OUR STORIES
TOLD BY US

Celebrating the
African contribution
to the UK HIV response

First published in 2023 by ZZUK Press
www.zzuk.org

Copy edited by Julia Thorley

Cover and inside illustration by Charity Nyirenda

Design and layout by Jane Shepherd

ISBN 978-1-7394622-1-5

This book is our labour of love, our gift to you. We are honouring those living with and affected by HIV in the African communities in the UK.

At times you may feel unheard and unseen, hidden under a veil of stigma – we hear you, we see you; your stories are important and continue to shape history. Never give up on your dreams – you matter!

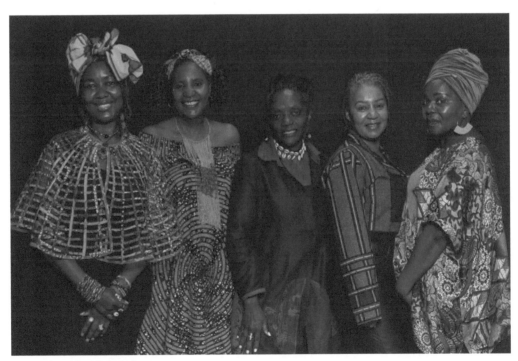

Photography © Sokari. IG @sokarieu

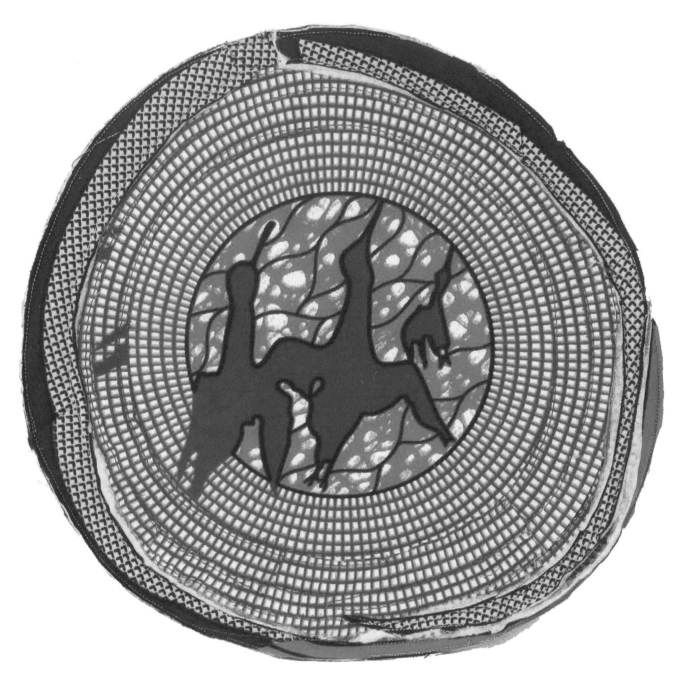

Fabric design from Ghana, Ahenfei/Abusua/Ayawa, meaning unity.

OUR STORIES TOLD BY US

Celebrating the African contribution to the UK HIV response

Angelina Namiba
Charity Nyirenda
Memory Sachikonye
Rebecca Mbewe
Winnie Ssanyu Sseruma

CONTENTS

9 **Foreword**
Winnie Byanyima

11 **Editors' introduction: why this book and why now?**

15 **Creating a vision to symbolise our journey**
Charity Nyirenda

AUTHOR CONTRIBUTIONS

18 **The language of HIV: ubuntu – we are who we are because of others**
Angelina Namiba

30 **Volunteer? Me? Why? Making sense of life experiences**
Charity Nyirenda

38 **The wedding and winter that changed my life: the silence of HIV**
Memory Sachikonye

47 **Behind closed doors**
Rebecca Mbewe

56 **HIV found me and altered my life in ways that I never knew were possible**
Winnie Ssanyu Sseruma

66 **If You Need Me**
Group poem

EXPERIENCES OF PEOPLE LIVING WITH HIV

68 **A cup of tea and a diagnosis of HIV: responding to my HIV diagnosis**
Adela Senkubuge

72 **Unlearning life: the touchstone of how HIV care should be provided**
Alice Welbourn

80 **Creative ways to convey messages: trying to change the HIV stigma story**
Bakita Kasadha

85 **Welcome to my world of living with HIV: this is my journey of living positively, openly and fabulously**
Bisi Alimi

89 **Navigating HIV and adolescence: a home away from home**
Bryan Dramiga

95 **Volunteering to support myself: the hidden disease of others**
Eunice Sinyemu

96 **Fight on comrades!**
Fernando Monteiro

102 **Evidence of a sinful life: accessing information to highlight the truth about HIV**
Godwyns Onwuchekwa

109 **Balancing rocks**
Jane Shepherd

112 **Queer folks: finding the right community for me**
Jide Macaulay

115 **Failure to thrive: the devastating effects of HIV in the Zimbabwe community**
Lazarus Mungure

120 **The sky is the limit: grieving for the loss of my old life**
Laura Dayit

124 **Hitting the ground running: processing my HIV diagnosis through empathising with others**
Marc Thompson

130 **There is no life before HIV: growing up living with HIV**
Mercy Shibemba

132 **Dreams, ambitions and a diagnosis of HIV**
Neo Moepi

134 **Bent, not broken: living positively and dying with dignity**
Noerine Kaleeba

141 **I knew I was different, just didn't know what it was called: 'Young man are you a homosexual?'**
Shaun Mellors

148 **The rise of the feminine power: the beauty and energy of African cultures**
Silvia Petretti

151 **The art of writing about HIV: campaigning for social change**
Simon Collins

160 **Sex in the suburbs: a desire to do something more meaningful with my life**
Susan Cole-Haley

165 **Common threads: a professional and personal journey**
Tristan Barber

172 **Today I**
Group poem

ALLIES

174 **Engineering HIV prevention: the grassroots approach**
Badru Male

179 **Would you like to be a doctor? I can help people stay well in different ways**
Chamut Kifetew

182 **An afterthought from Zimbabwe to London: falling into HIV care**
Charles Mazhude

186 **Suicide, stigma and a passion to fight HIV-related stigma**
Cheikh Traore

191 **All aboard: the anger and passion in HIV activism**
Elisabeth Crafer

196 **An accidental HIV activist: science, research and ensuring representation**
Ibi Fakoya

201 **The right people in the right place at the right time**
Jane Anderson

205 **My reflections on and journey through the HIV/AIDS pandemic: A public health perspective**
Professor Kevin Fenton

211 **From London to Malawi: caring for communities affected by HIV**
Mas Chaponda

215 **'AIDS: Don't Die of Ignorance'– the stories that shape you**
Michelle Croston

218 **The joy of working in HIV and the people you meet along the way**
Nneka Nwokolo

222 **The black community needs a voice: an intoxicating mix of anger, passion, hope and desire**
Priscilla Nkwenti

227 **From a conservative Christian background to a world of HIV activism and faith**
Rev Ije Ajibade

231 **Following a dream: in pursuit of a career in HIV medicine**
Sanjay Bhagani

234 **Having the privilege of working in HIV care**
Vanessa Apea

238 **Their shoes could fit my feet: supporting real people**
Vernal Scott

240 **This Summer**
Group poem

241 **Postcards to a different version of me**

248 **If I had magic wand I would want ...** Group wishes

251 **Acronyms**

252 **Organisations**

254 **Studies**

255 **Acknowledgements**

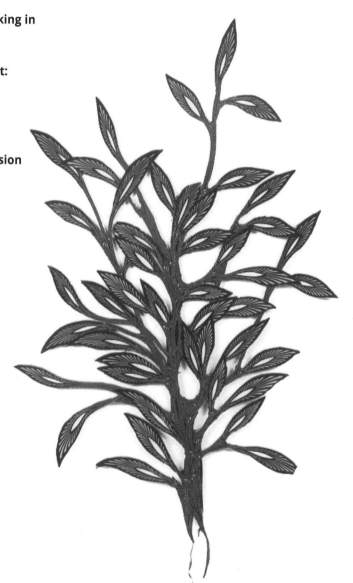

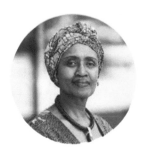

FOREWORD

Winnie Byanyima, Executive Director, Joint United Nations Programme on HIV/AIDS (UNAIDS), Under-Secretary-General of the United Nations

 Our Stories Told By Us is a remarkable collection of stories, primarily from Africans living with HIV who, in the early days of the AIDS pandemic, were able to access antiretroviral medicines in the UK that were unavailable in Africa.

These moving stories give a human face to a great injustice: the denial of HIV treatment for ten long years for people living in Africa – because medicines that were saving lives in rich countries were priced far beyond the reach of people in the developing countries.

Most contributors in this collection represent a migration of Africans who were born, already living or migrated to Europe and North America seeking better opportunities to change their lives, including women seeking greener pastures to raise their children. They came from communities being devastated by AIDS and settled in a country where new drugs were offering hope.

Many Africans will see their lives and those of their loved-ones retold in these pages. I certainly did. I was moved by the courage of each and every contributor in the face of so much loss and uncertainty, and equally struck by their strength, dignity and resilience. I was uplifted by the richness of the African diaspora; its strength, compassion and humour. Each story is a beautiful testimony of the power of individual agency and the collective action of communities.

By gathering these first-hand accounts of African migrants in the UK, the authors have brought to light an important moment in the history of the HIV pandemic, that is seldom told.

Our Stories Told By Us reminds us that we are stronger when we all stand together. But the book also reminds us that stigma is still alive and well, despite the progress made over the past 40 years, despite the best efforts of so many people, including those featured here, to change perceptions about people living with HIV.

Angelina Namiba writes, "We still don't have a pill to treat stigma."

But I say to her and her fellow co-authors, Charity Nyirenda, Memory Sachikonye, Rebecca Mbewe and Winnie Ssanyu Sseruma – we may not have a pill to treat stigma. But you have given us the gift of this book. The first of its kind to showcase the voices, lives, and leadership of Africans living with HIV in the UK, it will go a long way to combating stigma and discrimination.

I hope this book is read by many, both within the African diaspora and beyond. It is a moving tribute to the strength of the human spirit, to community activism and to love.

EDITORS' INTRODUCTION: WHY THIS BOOK AND WHY NOW?

As the editors and authors, we would like to start this book with some thought-provoking statistics. HIV has been on a rampage across the globe for nearly 40 years, but unless you are living with it, affected by it, work on HIV or related issues, or are interested in some way, shape or form, like many others you could be forgiven for thinking that Covid-19 is the worst pandemic we have had to deal with in the last half-century.

To date, just under 40 million people around the world are currently living with HIV, and almost the same number have died from HIV-related ailments in the last four decades.

The majority of people living with HIV are on HIV treatment and living longer, not dying, and that is why, in part, there are nearly 40 million of us. The lifesaving HIV treatments, though not perfect for all, are something to be really grateful for, but not everyone around the world is able to access these treatments. This remains a source of great frustration and an area of increased activism.

Currently, the global HIV goals are; access to HIV treatment for everyone who needs it, the majority of people living with HIV to have an HIV test and be diagnosed, for those on treatment to have achieved viral suppression, and for no new HIV infections by 2030. There other targets that many of us living with HIV and involved in the HIV sector would like to see, including, continuing to address HIV-related stigma, achieving good quality of life and so much more. You may ask yourself, are these targets achievable? Yes, they are! However, are we going to achieve them by 2030? Unlikely. The most logical question is, why? There are a number of factors preventing this from happening. A major reason is inequalities – the global theme for World AIDS Day 2022. Inequalities keep us from ending HIV, and has become a subject of much discussion and narrative within the HIV sector. This is captured well in the following quote by Winnie Byanyima, Executive

Director of UNAIDS: *"What world leaders need to do is crystal clear. In one word: equalise. Equalise access to rights, equalise access to services, equalise access to the best science and medicine. Equalising will not only help the marginalised. It will help everyone."*

This book focuses on the UK HIV epidemic, and within that reflects on the HIV experience of African communities through individual stories and reflections rather than HIV statistics. This is the first book specifically to do that. This has been made possible as a result of five Black African women living with HIV and residing in the UK.

However, it is important to highlight briefly what the HIV epidemic looks like in the UK, especially for those who might not be familiar with the subject matter. The most affected communities are men who have sex with men, bisexual men and people from African communities. The majority of Africans living with HIV live in London, most identify as heterosexual, but not exclusively. There are more African women living with HIV than African men. The majority of children and young people under the age of 18 who are living with HIV in the UK are of African descent.

Despite Covid-19-related challenges in assessing HIV data between 2019 and 2022, the UK 2021 data shows that the number of people testing for HIV and living with HIV and in care is returning to pre-Covid-19 levels. However, there are differences among population groups. While there has been an increase in HIV testing among many groups since 2019, especially online testing, the number of heterosexual men taking tests continued to fall. The number of new HIV diagnoses continued to fall in London but plateaued outside. Heterosexual men and women seem to be accessing HIV testing less than other groups and this is a concern. Finally, there is still a high level of unawareness of HIV pre-exposure prophylaxis (PrEP), higher numbers of late diagnoses, and weaker indications of recovery among heterosexual males and heterosexual and bisexual females.

There are plenty of HIV epidemiological data on African communities in the UK and most of it makes for challenging reading, showing that there is still a lot of work to do. But improvements also continue, thanks to people from African communities, allies, health personnel and support from the government and charity sectors. What this book aims to reflect on are the individual stories of recovery, resilience and leadership in the HIV response in the UK – stories we don't normally read about. This is the first book of its kind to explore the contribution African individuals and communities have made to the fight against HIV. In this important period of reflection on over 40 years of the UK's HIV response, we felt it was critical to tell these stories. Above all else, it was pivotal for Africans living with HIV to lead this project and to tell our own stories in our own words. If not now, then when? If not us, then who?

None of us had ever compiled a book before or written our own stories. The driving ambitions for embarking on this project were to amplify unheard voices and record this social history, a history that, so far, has been absent from the HIV story in the UK. As the enormity of the task began to dawn on us, we had to think more pragmatically than emotionally. We had to bring on board partners to work with, there was fundraising to do, and finding the stories (from communities notoriously known to avoid talking about difficult issues, especially HIV). We wanted to create an inclusive project, so we needed allies to build a comprehensive picture of the African HIV experience and so much more, but at no point did any of us think that we couldn't do this. We just kept tapping into the healthy network of contacts we have built over the years, and they did not disappoint us. We have been even more empowered by the wave of goodwill we have received through working on this project.

We approached Positive East to hold any funds we raised and to support with project management. Mark Santos, Executive Director, welcomed the project with open arms and sat in on the monthly meetings. Michelle Croston, nurse, associate professor and author, was exceptional in supporting us with the first edits of the stories. We then talked to various people with expertise in writing, took writing and poetry workshops, approached web and book designers and crucially, contributors of the stories, to make sure we had the content for the book.

We offered contributors some guiding questions that they were free to answer or not. Most of them replied in writing while a few asked for an oral interview.

- Tell us about your life before diagnosis or before you joined the HIV sector.
- What drew you to get involved?
- Describe the HIV landscape when you first got involved or diagnosed.
- What have been your personal highs and lows and any African community highs and contributions?
- What relationships have had the most meaning for you? What has helped?

- What are some of the lessons learned and what can be done differently, particularly in relation to African communities?
- If you could go back in time what advice would you give your younger self? What advice would you give to your future self?
- What are some of your key achievements and/or contributions to the sector?
- If you had a magic wand, what would you wish for?

Collecting the stories was never going to be easy, but no matter how difficult it got, we were clear with everyone that there was to be no anonymity (tough, but necessary). We are confronting HIV stigma head on. It is about standing with heads held high, taking back our agency as individuals and communities, and reflecting on our contribution towards the UK's goal of ending HIV transmission by 2030.

In this book, we have shared some of our experiences and the reflections of many more people like us, and, together with our allies, we hope the world never forgets what we went through, what we did and how we lived, fighting for our very survival as HIV and the stigma related to it threatened our lives. Our hope is that this project is a foundation that African communities can build on and continue to document the journeys of the African diaspora, highlighting the positive impact we are making in other areas in the UK, rather than always focusing on our challenges.

This project has three phases. The first was to gather content, which we have successfully achieved. The second is to turn this book into a digital resource that can be accessed by a wider audience. The final phase is a UK roadshow, talking to African communities in different regions about how to continue to address the impact of HIV on the African diaspora, but above all else, how to support people with HIV to live well and achieve their full potential. For this part, we hope to see you in the audience as we celebrate the wonderful stories we have shared.

When we came up with this idea, and as we continue to see the project through, we want to encourage those living with HIV to embrace their lives and live unapologetically. Through learning, asking for support and supporting each other, we have achieved far more than we ever dreamed of. We believe in action, doing and not talking. We want to continue to drive the change we want to see, to lead but also bring others with us. The journey continues. We look forward to seeing you along the way.

CREATING A VISION TO SYMBOLISE OUR JOURNEY

Charity Nyirenda

When we first started this project, I had so many ideas swirling in my head. I could see lots of African colours, fabrics, patterns, but not just any pattern. I wanted them to mean something, to be entwined, symbolising all our journeys, experiences, our growth, strength, unity, freedom and hope. I wanted the design to capture the uniqueness of the African experience. It was important to me that we create a bold and vibrant collage in the book. The edges of the fabric are purposefully frayed, symbolising the challenges and imperfections of communities. But we continue to work for unity

The cover design

The cover of the book uses a tree, the map of Africa and the power of sun. The tree is an oasis of peace symbolising strength, growth, stability, standing tall against all weathers. For me, this is representative of how we stand together against the discrimination and stigma of living with HIV. This tree motif is from a Côte d'Ivoire pattern called 'grotto', meaning social recognition. The idea was that the tree would represent all our shared stories, each leaf representing a story. As the tree grows upwards and outwards, it is symbolic of our bodies and minds growing, expanding, increasing with knowledge. The networks of branches represent our interconnectedness and the multiple generations living with and affected by HIV. Within the design and reflective of life each tree is unique, just like us, which represents the uniqueness of our stories; but there is also a sense of togetherness and a reminder that, like trees, we are never alone or isolated, but we are connected via our roots to the world and to each other in some way.

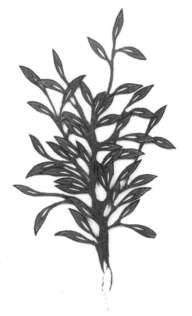

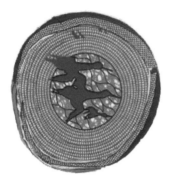

The book is about African people telling their stories about living with HIV in the UK. To represent this, I chose red and black fabric, symbolising blood and race that connects us, the red dots being our steps or journeys, connecting us. As we grow, the twining roots continue. Africa is the hottest continent in the world, so within the book I have used brilliant yellow for the sun, as it changes the direction of light, heat and energy as it travels across Africa and the rest of the world. The image of the sun also indicates the cycle of life from birth to adulthood to death and rebirth.

The fabric with overlapping birds is called Ahenfei/Abusua/Ayawa in Ghana, meaning unity. In unity we stand together as one. The birds represent our families, community, allies and the support around us, flocking together in waves. These symbolise the power, force and energy we all have within us. It brings constant change and flexibility, which we have all experienced when living with HIV.

Calmness, purification, washing away the past and renewing our souls

Each page in this book has an African pattern that connects to the next page through to the end of the book.

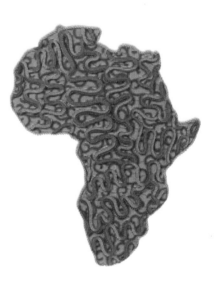

I felt so blessed when you asked me to create a canvas for you to see your stories. They're in artistic form, a backdrop, a backdrop to our lives, so all colours, patterns and fabrics used give me ideas that I could use. It was our journeys, our stories, I portrayed on every page, the tree, the map, the sun, the waves, the land and town as symbols saved, the links to homes, our motherland. We are woven by our loving hands. Our journeys have been sometimes harsh. But both bond us now, just like a cast performing in some kind of play. Yes, now fight. We are here to stay.

AUTHOR CONTRIBUTIONS

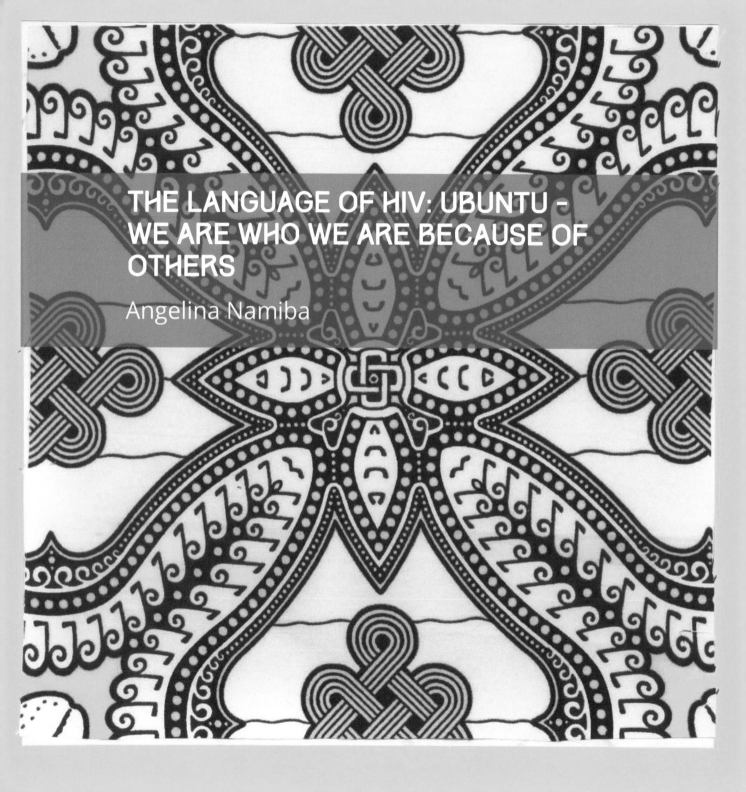

THE LANGUAGE OF HIV: UBUNTU – WE ARE WHO WE ARE BECAUSE OF OTHERS

Angelina Namiba

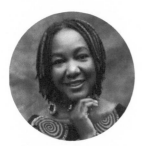

was born in Kenya, on 17th March 1967, St Patrick's Day. My parents separated shortly after I was born. Their divorce was in the papers because at the time it was quite a big deal for a woman to divorce her husband and get custody of the children. Shortly after they separated, my dad moved to Tanzania and my mum, then a social worker with the Kenya Prisons Service, got a scholarship from the Israel School of Social Work, to go and study in Swansea in Wales. She decided to leave us with a series of friends and relatives, and sent money monthly for our upkeep.

We later moved to Tanzania to live with my dad. After a few years, Dad took a transfer back to Kenya and we settled in Mombasa, where I finished my primary school education, as well as my secondary school. For high school I went to a boarding school in Kitui, a small town in Eastern Kenya.

After my A-levels, I went back to Mombasa, where I first worked as a shop assistant for one of the curio/tourist shops on the popular Moi Avenue, one of the main streets in Mombasa. I then moved on to work at the Kenya Marine and Fisheries Research Institute as an Information Officer in its library.

After a couple of years, Mum suggested that I apply for university in the UK so I could join her. She had by then finished her studies and was living and working in London as a social worker with Hackney Social Services.

I went to the local British Council in Mombasa, was given some UCAS (the clearing house) application forms and made the application to come and study Librarianship. In May 1989, I upped sticks and moved to London to join Mum and go to university. In September 1989, I started my course in Information Technology and Library Management at the now Manchester Metropolitan University.

In my final year as I was doing my exams, I got very ill. I was so poorly I could barely get out of bed. When I finally managed to drag myself to the GP, he asked me if I had looked in the mirror. I told him I was so ill that the last thing I thought of was looking in the mirror. He asked me to look in the mirror in the surgery and all I could see was just yellow. I was quite jaundiced to say the least.

He sent me for a test at the local hospital. Because I was doing my finals and left for London soon after, I didn't find out what it was I had until the family GP in London called me to his surgery and told me that I had had hepatitis B. He then asked me to go for an HIV test. That was quite a shock for me. HIV was not anything I had thought about in relation to me, but it was even more scary for me because not that long before my brother Kennedy, whom we nicknamed K, had just told us that he had HIV. Unfortunately, it was the pre-HAART (highly active anti-retroviral treatment) era, so he spent a lot of time in and out of hospital and the London Lighthouse and Mildmay hospices. He also had meningitis, Karposi's sarcoma (a type of cancer) and epileptic fits. Sadly, he died a year later of AIDS-related pneumocystis pneumonia (PCP).

So when the GP asked me to go for an HIV test it was quite challenging for me to deal with it. Apart from watching my brother slowly die, all I saw around me in relation to HIV was negativity, and images of people who were emaciated, ill, dying. The GP gave me a piece of paper with instructions on it for me to go for an HIV test at Whipps Cross Hospital. I took the piece of paper, went home, hid it under my bed and went to the local library to look up hepatitis B. I wanted nothing to do with HIV. I didn't go for the test.

After a couple of weeks, I received a letter from the GP strongly suggesting that I go for a test. I remember the word strongly was underlined. It scared me so much that I went for the test, but I didn't go back for the result. In fact, I never went back to that GP's surgery. (With hindsight of course I am grateful that he asked me to go for the test, because if I hadn't found out about my status then I wouldn't be here today.)

After a little while, the GP sent me a package that included a list of information about places that did pre-test and post-test counselling. I went to a local one, had some counselling, re-did the test and this time I was better prepared so went back for my result.

It came back positive. I was only 25 years old.

Because I was much more prepared for the result, I knew I had to make a choice about what to do. Luckily for me, I got my diagnosis in almost the same week as I got an offer for a job as Information Officer at the then South Thames Regional Health Authority. (Prior to that I had been working as a waitress to make ends meet whilst I looked for a job). I decided to take the job whilst I waited to die. I figured it was better than sitting in my room staring miserably at the walls. With hindsight, that was one of the best decisions I made back then, because I believe working, along with other positive things that happened in my life then, is what helped me cope and has kept me going to the present day.

Peer support helped me to cope

One day out of the blue, one of my friends said to me, 'Angelina, I have something to tell you.' I asked her what it was and she said, 'I have HIV.'

Yes! I thought to myself, because up to that point I thought I was the only woman in London living with HIV. But here was another woman, here in London, and she just happened to be my friend. I hadn't been able to tell anyone, including my family, about my diagnosis. (I had only been able to tell my very close friend Cicy. We went to secondary school together in Kenya). I told her when I went for the second test and rang her after I got my result, and she was very supportive and has remained so. I straight away told my friend about my diagnosis, and she proceeded to take me to a support group where I met five other women living with HIV. One was a mum, one was working, they were all just leading regular lives. Meeting those women gave me the drive and motivation to continue living.

Once I had received the peer support I needed, I decided to volunteer in the HIV sector. When I saw a job advertised at Positively Women for an African Client Services Co-ordinator to work with women living with HIV, I applied and got the job. So began my journey of volunteering and working in the HIV sector. The peer support I received was invaluable and I felt that I needed to give back what I had received and to support other women in my position in coping with their diagnosis and moving on with their lives.

Freddie Mercury dies of AIDS: the doom and gloom of living with HIV

When I was diagnosed, the HIV landscape was pretty much a lot of doom and gloom. A lasting image in my mind from that time was a picture of Freddie Mercury on the front page of one of the red top newspapers with the caption, 'Freddie Mercury dies of AIDS' or something along those lines. There was a lot of negativity connected to HIV. Many people diagnosed at that time were given six months to live. The only treatment available to treat us at the time was AZT and other earlier toxic drugs that had some really terrible and very visible side effects, including darkening of the skin and fingernails and toenails, anaemia and lipodystrophy (redistribution of fat away from the legs and buttocks to the stomach and other areas). These were so pronounced that I remember once asking a lady who had come to the support group, when she was due, and her telling me that she wasn't pregnant, that it was a side effect of the HIV medication she was taking. I never asked anybody that question again, unless they had expressly told me that they were pregnant. Unlike today where people take just one pill or two once a day (and we have reached a point where a monthly or bi-monthly injection is available), in those days people took a cocktail of drugs, 20 or 30 pills a day, many of them toxic, some of them with food restrictions. Some of them had to be stored in the fridge. These were all barriers to people adhering to their treatment, but they needed to in order to stay alive.

There was a lot of fear both directed at and from us as people living with HIV. Watching my own brother getting ill and dying in front of me was really challenging, because I could see my own life panning out ahead of me. We lost a lot of friends and colleagues along the way. I remember a time when there were funerals weekly and sometimes you had to choose which one to go to. There were that many.

Then there was also the stigma, myths and misconceptions about HIV, which sadly still persist today, some 40 years into the epidemic. We have certainly come a long way in terms of how treatments for HIV have developed, to a point where if someone adheres to their treatment – takes their treatment as advised and follows any restrictions, which are very few nowadays – and if they achieve and maintain an undetectable viral load, it means they cannot pass HIV onto their sexual partner or their unborn child. This is also known as U=U, Undetectable=Untransmittable.

There has been fantastic progress in terms of the science. Unfortunately, stigma hasn't caught up. Stigma prevents people from testing for HIV, and from accessing and staying engaged in the lifesaving health and social care services that they need to stay well.

However, a lot of progress has been made and a lot more can be done in terms of challenging and addressing stigma from an individual, community and societal level. This needs to be done in collaboration with all the main stakeholders; people living with HIV, health and social care providers, the media, faith leaders, governments, funders, allies, the public, and those not living with HIV. The list is endless. Challenging and addressing stigma is not just the responsibility of activists and advocates living with HIV. We all have a role to play. People do not exist in a vacuum. For me, this is perfectly embodied in the South African Zulu term ubuntu (in full, ubuntu kubuntu kabantu), which means we are who we are because of others. It has the basic qualities of compassion and humility.

The good news is that we have moved on. There are now many more people living with HIV who can act as role models, giving voice and visibility to their peers; there are religious and other institutions (INERELA+ and others), and sections of the media that are sharing facts and not fear about HIV. We are also calling for a change in the language that we use to talk about and describe HIV and those who live with it, including lots of campaigns that highlight the positive aspects of living with HIV such as Positive Affirmation Day, More than HIV, Can't pass it on, and so many others. The UNAIDS call for a focus on global solidarity and shared responsibility for World AIDS Day 2021 is so apt right now and should be continued yearly as we move forwards.

Coming into contact with my people: working out what people think

There have been lows but also many highs on my journey of living with and working in the HIV sector. The lows include losing many family, friends and colleagues along the journey to AIDS-related illnesses. The lows also include seeing and coming into contact with many people, particularly women, who have still not come to terms with their diagnosis, who are still self-stigmatising, who are still in the denial about their status; who have put their lives on hold and will not have relationships or even think about starting families; who limit their lives and relationships to only being around other people living with HIV; who are more concerned about what people think of them than they are about focusing on their health and wellbeing and living their best lives without letting HIV define who they are and dominating their lives; who are, understandably, incredibly afraid to share their HIV status, because they are emotionally and economically dependent on their partners and significant others, such that for them telling others about their status can lead to them losing their homes; who endure and stay in abusive relationships because they believe or are made to believe that no one will love them because of their HIV. My ethos about people who shun you or treat you negatively because you have HIV is to ask, of what benefit are they to my life? Do they pay my rent? Feed me and my child? Pay my bills? Do anything for me? If the answer to those questions is no, then they can take a walk, but I am acutely aware of the fact that I am in a privileged position where I have a home to go to and I have food on my table, and even if I didn't, I am lucky to have a great network of family and friends around to support me and whom I can go to in times of need. And so, I continue to be open about my status, because I believe it is important that those of us who can be safely and publicly open about our status continue to do so in order to carry on challenging the myths, misconceptions and stigma that still exist around HIV today.

On a societal level, there have been many highs. These include watching the HIV landscape change in terms of treatment development to an extent where now most people only need a pill or two a day, and will soon have access to a monthly injection and other innovative ways of taking medication that will make it easier for those not able to adhere to the daily regime for whatever reason; the fact that treatment now has the potential to transform lives in that U=U means people living with HIV cannot pass HIV on to their sexual partners or their unborn child; the fact that guidelines for the management of HIV in pregnancy have changed such that women living with HIV can now give birth vaginally and only need to have caesarean section in an emergency, like other women not living with HIV; that mothers living with HIV who chose to breastfeed can be supported to do so safely.

On a personal level, highs include getting access to peer support so early on in my diagnosis; learning to cope with and live well with HIV; getting the opportunity to volunteer and work in the HIV sector and to give back what helped me not just to survive but also to thrive; meeting many women, children, young people, who trusted me and let me into their lives, and enriched my life along the way; the many colleagues and friends I have met on the journey; the opportunities I have had to develop personally, to learn new skills such as group facilitation, public speaking, project management, creative writing; treatment advocacy; the opportunities to travel to conferences and other forums to meet and network and learn and share, and meet celebrities and other important/key players; and the opportunity to be involved in setting up the 4M Network of Mentor Mothers, with an amazing team of women (friends and colleagues) living with HIV.

Flaws and all: nurturing the relationships that matter most

During my HIV journey, so many relationships have helped me and all have a lot of meaning for me. These include the counsellor who supported me through accepting the fact that I needed to go for the HIV test as advised by the GP, who gave me the strength to accept and deal with my positive diagnosis; my friend Cecilia who was on the other end of the line when I went for the test and after I got my results, and who continues to be an incredible source of support, strength and friendship; my friend L who trusted me enough to tell me about her own HIV status and who enabled me to open up about mine, and who linked me into the peer support that saved my life; to my family, my late mum and dad, brothers, sisters, nieces and nephews, in-laws – the list goes on – who accepted me and continue to love and support me and have not been fazed by my HIV diagnosis; friends and colleagues living with HIV who have supported me in my work and shaped my journey over the years, and enabled me to grow; activists, advocates and colleagues in HIV community organisations; numerous HIV clinicians and colleagues within the pharmaceutical industry, who have shaped supported and given me opportunities to enable my advocacy and to reach many and to thrive in my work; all the women and young people, and a some men living with HIV whom I have had the privilege to meet and support over the years, who have trusted me and allowed me into their lives, who have and continue to give me the drive to do the work that I do; my close-knit group of friends, too many to mention, but in particular my ZZUK sisters Rebecca, Charity, Memory and Winnie, who have seen me through a lot and who remain a constant in my life; and last but by no means least, my beautiful, talented, caring and loving daughter Malika Hamzaa, who is my reason for living, who has and who continues to love and accept me for who I am, flaws and all.

The reality of some of the lessons that I have learnt

Some of the lessons learnt along the way include the fact/reality that:

Successful responses respect human rights. Gender inequalities that fuel the epidemic must be addressed. Health inequalities must be anticipated, acknowledged and addressed. HIV is increasingly concentrated among poor people and countries and more vulnerable populations. Interventions must take account of this. No one-size model or intervention fits all. Empowering and enabling young people is essential to bring the end of the epidemic forward.

Prevention methods, lifesaving treatments, and the results of scientific breakthroughs in prevention and care must be made broadly available on an equitable and affordable basis for all. Treatments should be made available to all no matter where they live. It is important to alleviate the social and economic impact.

Responding to the epidemic requires effective measures to support risk reduction and reduce social and economic vulnerability. Strategies that systematically promote social inclusion, extend access to information, essential services and supportive legal and social norms can overcome vulnerability and help overcome the impact of the epidemic. Medication for HIV and opportunistic infections and infrastructures, training and availability of resources, medication and social care system must be made available. Care and treatment should be comprehensive.

National governments, working with civil society, must provide leadership and means to ensure that national and international efforts respond to country and community needs. Political leadership matters. Early in the epidemic, political leadership was glaringly absent. Many heads of state refused to acknowledge the existence of the virus. Helping fuel stigma and thwarting efforts to promote prevention and behaviour change. In countries like the USA, it took activists and activist groups like ACT who made noise and catalysed change and to force leaders to step up.

People living with HIV and affected by HIV must be meaningfully engaged, involved, supported and properly funded in their efforts to address the epidemic. Successful responses have their roots in the community. That community advocacy is incredibly important and key. As an example, in 1987 in the USA, HIV largely affected gay men and received little public attention. Gay advocacy groups such as ACT UP mobilised around AIDS. They targeted pharmaceutical company Burroughs Wellcome for high prices of the drug AZT and the Food and Drug Administration (FDA) for its drug access and approval policies. Subsequently, pharma lowered the price of AZT and the FDA regulations rapidly evolved to improve drug access and allow surrogate end points in clinical trial of ARVs. A decade later, TAC (Treatment Access Campaign) worked to increase access to ARVs in South Africa. The engagement of affected communities for both their insights and advocacy will continue to be needed in the fight against HIV.

There is no pill for stigma

Knowledge is power and we need effective health communication and information. Spread facts not fear. We have a fantastic range of treatments that enable people living with HIV to lead regular lives. We also now have the concept of U=U. However, we still haven't got a pill to tackle stigma and this is what is killing our communities. More efforts therefore need to be put into addressing self and societal stigma in order that we can reach a point whereby we have zero new infections, zero HIV-related deaths and zero HIV-related stigma. It is important to note, too, that the concept of U=U alone will not solve the issue of stigma. We need a comprehensive set of holistic services and ongoing research into all the relevant treatment and prevention methods in order for us to reach the UNAIDS 95-95-95 targets, not forgetting the fourth 95, quality of life, because people living with HIV are more than an undetectable viral load. We have lives.

Champagne and celebration moments

Achievements and contributions have been spread over the years and over a number of HIV charities and organisations, including: speaking at numerous local, national and international conferences on issues relating to women and HIV; co-authoring numerous papers, including The language of HIV: a guide for nurses; volunteering for lots of different initiatives and community organisations, including the Children's HIV Association (CHIVA); being a lay member of Royal College of Obstetricians and Gynaecologists (RCOG) Women's Voices; World Health Organization (WHO) working groups; GNP+; S.A.F.E. Kenya; being publicly open about my status in print and on radio, TV and online media in order to raise the visibility and voice of women living with HIV, as well as challenge the myths, misconceptions and stigmas that still surround HIV today; training mentoring and skilling up women and young people living with HIV to soar.

Organisations I have been involved in:

- **Body and Soul Charity** – Volunteer and founding member and one of the first members of the first board of trustees.
- **Positively Women** – One of two first African Client services co-ordinator tasked with, amongst other things, encouraging African women living with HIV to access services. As Project Manager led on the Taking Part Project, training mentoring and upskilling women living with HIV (many of them African and who have gone on to do great things), and promoting their involvement in forming and informing local and national strategy and policy.
- **AHPN (African HIV Policy Network)** – As programme lead for NAHIP, a national HIV prevention programme working with African community organisations to provide a range of HIV prevention interventions and structural services; led on the development of Life and Knowledge Muslim toolkit for faith leaders. Also led on

the development and delivery of The Knowledge, the Will and the Power: a plan of action to meet the HIV prevention needs of Africans living in England.

- **Positively UK** – Project manager for the Primary Care Access project, a research project working with the HIV community, HIV clinicians, GPs and HIV commissioners, aimed at recommending models of care to enable patients with HIV to access their GP services – co-authored the report: Primary Care Access: How General Practice Can Better Respond to the Needs of People Living with HIV. Also, led on setting up From Pregnancy to Baby and Beyond, a one-year pilot project aimed at developing an effective and sustainable model of education, information, emotional and practical support for three target groups of women living with HIV, namely women diagnosed HIV positive antenatally, women having babies after an HIV diagnosis and those considering having babies. This project was the first of its kind in the UK.

- **HIV i-Base** – Trained as a treatment advocate and provided training and timely HIV treatment information to people living with HIV and healthcare professionals.

- **Salamander Trust** – Led on the planning development and delivery of the 4M Training of Trainers for women living with HIV. Including the 4M Network of Mentor Mothers living with HIV. Led on the writing and development of a training guided based on the above. Led on the planning, development and delivery of the 4M perinatal peer mentoring project with women living with HIV, across eight regions of the UK, and on the planning, development and delivery of the same model of the 4M project (4M+) in four regions of Kenya and Uganda. Trained as a facilitator for the Stepping Stones with Children programme. A programme designed for use with children affected by HIV, aged 5–8, 9–14 and their caregivers.

- **4M Network of Mentor Mothers living with HIV** – co-founder, member and many achievements over the years.

Maximise your time on earth, tomorrow is not promised.

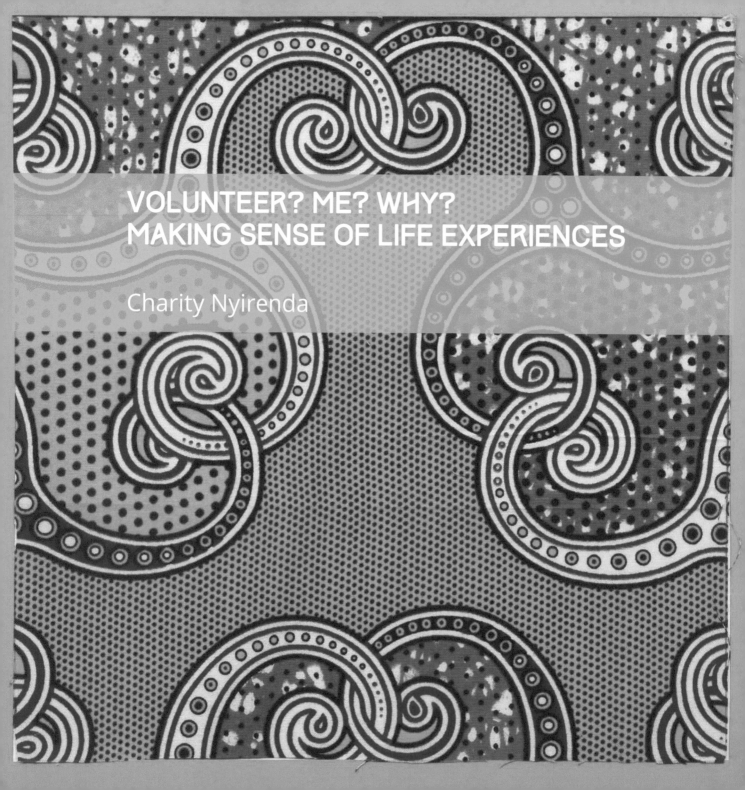

VOLUNTEER? ME? WHY?
MAKING SENSE OF LIFE EXPERIENCES

Charity Nyirenda

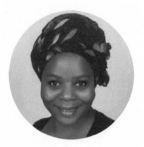

'm originally from Zambia. I was raised in a middle-class home and had my education in Zambia. After my college I worked as a receptionist for a German company where I made friends outside my family background. Socialising with different people of other backgrounds made me understand life from a different perspective. The knowledge I acquired at the German company enabled a friend, who worked for a government organisation, to find me a job at a printing firm where I worked as a copy typist. My work experience exposed me to the opportunity of travelling outside Zambia. I had a thought of visiting the UK, which I discussed with my parents and was encouraged to do so, if I wished. I was very outgoing, which made people not see the shyness part of me. I took a bold step in leaving my comfort zone to visit the UK, which ended up being a migration. Upon arrival in the UK, I observed a different style of life (culture, weather, food, organised means of transportation and idea of leisure), which I adopted very quickly and I felt I could cope with settling in UK. I enrolled in studies while I worked part-time. Since then, I have settled in England, though I had what seems to a shortcoming in my life when I was diagnosed HIV positive. As time went on, I learnt to live well with HIV.

Being diagnosed with HIV in 2003 changed my life. I felt isolated and not worthy. I was referred to Positively UK (formerly known as Positively Women) as a service user in 2007. After a few months I was asked if I could apply to be a volunteer caseworker. This came as a shock to me, because it never occurred to me that I could volunteer and not be paid. To be honest, my answer was, why? At this time, I had immigration issues, and not being allowed to work made me feel useless, with no purpose in life.

Days later I decided to have a go. I undertook relevant volunteer training about the organisation. I received a great deal of peer support from Positively UK and from friends I had made through volunteering. I would very much like to carry on volunteering, as I feel this gives me some purpose in life and stops me from feeling isolated.

Volunteering has taught me not to give up, to keep learning new skills and to support others affected by HIV. The staff who appreciate me will either encourage or pick me up if I'm down.

I'm thankful for the support I've received in all my struggles, because through it all I have learnt that I'm resilient. For that I am forever grateful, because I get back up again and again, which leads to self-realisation. Being welcomed with open arms by people around me, sharing my thoughts and experiences with others and being able to connect with and learn from people I have worked with has made volunteering one of the best decisions I have ever made!

I have learnt that volunteering can bring you into contact with all kinds of people from all walks of life, and can be a great way to learn new skills and share those I already have.

Positively UK provides peer-led support, advocacy and information to women, men and young people living with HIV to help them manage any aspect of their diagnosis, care and managing life with HIV. Working in partnership with the NHS, our peer work is integrated at clinics across London. Peer support services provided by volunteer peer mentors are an essential part of Positively UK's work.

I have been involved with Positively UK since 2007 and so understand the needs of people living with HIV and I'm able to support people at any stage of diagnosis, from recent diagnosis to wanting to start a family after diagnosis, to managing isolation.

Catwalk4Power

More recently, I have had a role as workshop facilitator and creative lead for Catwalk4Power, a peer support, arts empowerment and wellbeing project funded by Public Health England innovation Fund. This grant enabled us to coordinate three catwalks: one in London (on International Women's Day), the second in Brighton in collaboration with Sussex Beacon and Lunch Positive, and the third one in Manchester. It also attracted funding for three other performances and collaboration with The Royal Central School of Speech and Drama, and the Imperial College.

The final performance of Catwalk4Power, builds on a series of workshops (usually five): Leadership; Amazing bodies; Making sashes or clothes with key messages; Creative writing to craft spoken word for the performance; and a workshop for planning the performance. I was one of the founder members of this project and developed the workshops and performances until it was funded in January 2019.

I am extremely proud of the project as one of the founders. As a result of our success, we felt confident to take our message to an international stage. In March 2017 we hosted Catwalk4Power in Amsterdam. As a result of the work that I have carried out as a volunteer, I have learnt that in leading others you must learn to lead yourself.

Why do you want to have a test? Positive is good, right?

I decided to go and have an HIV test at St Anne's Hospital. I did not tell anyone about it because I did not want anyone to know that I had gone to the Sexual Health Clinic. Though I was confident to go to the clinic, I was scared, too, because I did not know what to expect. One of the nurses asked why I wanted to have the test done. I responded I was just curious. I was told to wait so they could explain what to expect. I was lucky enough to have pre and post-test counselling.

I had the test in December 2002. I had to wait for two weeks to get my result, but it felt like years to me. It was extremely stressful.

My HIV test results came back positive, and my understanding was that it was good result. The doctor had to explain to me what positive and negative meant when you are diagnosed. I just could not understand why positive meant something bad. I laughed so much and burst into tears. Being told about my diagnosis I was relieved: frustrated, obviously, but my overriding emotion was one of relief.

When the nurse explained everything, it just went in one ear and came out from the other. She told me so many things: how to protect myself and others, about medication and how it works, the side effects of medication and adherence. But I just sat through it and did not understand how this HIV thing worked. It was just too overwhelming. I was a mixture of emotions; one moment I was laughing and the next I was crying. Why did I get this thing? How did I get this thing?

I dealt with my diagnosis alone and the pain and depression I went through were unbearable. I did not absorb most of the things people were saying or talking about. It was a horrible feeling. I felt like I was trapped in the middle of this gigantic spider web and waiting to be poisoned by the spider and die. I was very much concerned about who to tell about my diagnosis. I wanted so much to tell my mother, but I could not because she was miles away. I did not tell anyone until after a few months. It was because I needed time to understand. My life became home, work, clinic. I would go to the clinic to get more information and support.

My journey started in January 2003 when I stepped out of the doctor's clinic and was diagnosed with HIV. So many questions were going through my head. Did I hear that right? I am going to die? No more sex? Does it mean I will never conceive?

At work it was difficult, because they put me on medication immediately, as my CD4 count (a measure of the body's immune functioning) was very low. I started with three ARVs and one for herpes. The side effects were horrible: my body swelled up, I had a rash on my face, my skin became very dark, my lips were dry, my hair became lifeless and I had scabs on my scalp. I felt terrible at the time.

I had nightmares for months, elephants chasing me in London! I would take the medication at night before I go to bed. I would just be there, very restless and unable to move. Going to the toilet was difficult. I would drop myself on the floor and drag myself or just pee there in a bowl. I could not stand or walk for the first month after I started taking the medication.

Is this normal?

There was one time when I forgot to take the meds in the evening, so I took it in the morning. Big mistake! On the bus on the way to work I felt sick. My phone kept dropping off my hand. I got off the bus and I was seeing triple vision of things around me. I don't know how I managed to get to Waitrose where I worked, but as soon as I did I fainted. The security guard caught me. I could hear people calling out my name, but I couldn't move or do anything. Afterwards, I recall someone asking me if I was on medication. I kept saying no, because I did not want them to know about my health.

I never took the medication in the morning again. But, let me tell you, it was the best HIV medicine I ever had in my life, aside from the first months, of course, when I was adjusting to it and later on when the effect of the drugs wearing off made me go to a dark place and felt tired all the time, which I wouldn't want to be again.

After six years I stopped taking it, even though it was also a great combination. It did wonders for me! You want to know? My chest became full, I became hyperactive and energetic. I remember one occasion I asked my consultant if it was normal that the medication kept me aroused all the time and he advised me that it was perfectly normal. The consultant told me I was lucky because some women would not get that! I became very adventurous. Once they changed the meds, everything became boring.

Sometimes I'm glad that I'm HIV positive and people think I'm weird when I say this. I think it's great, because if it were not for me living with HIV, I wouldn't be knowledgeable about this illness or about my health. Every time you go to the clinic, they check your health and if I was 'normal' I wouldn't know how my health is. I now have a wealth of knowledge about my levels of vitamin D, folic acids, CD4 count viral load, cholesterol, hepatitis. It has really helped me to look after my health now, and taught me so many things about living with HIV and how to look after yourself and others so that you don't transmit the virus.

I'm living well with HIV and trying to pursue my dreams, which I thought I would not be able to pursue when I was diagnosed. I'm living well, and although I still experience my dark moments at times I now know how to deal with them. I make sure I continue to support others living with HIV, because HIV and stigma are not over yet.

A prince among men: raising awareness

My highs have been being the poster girl/voice for people living with HIV and supporting the fight to combat the stigma and discrimination is still present by setting an example of how we can be strong, powerful, and proud even when we are living with HIV.

One of my highlights when raising awareness for HIV was when I made a Red Awareness brooch for Prince Harry, and I pinned it on him. Am I allowed to say more? I did ask him to unbutton two buttons so I could pin the brooch, which was bigger than the soft pin. All he said was, 'Please don't stab me,' and we all burst into laughter. He smelt so good. I could smell his aftershave all day!

The downsides of living with HIV have been when I've struggled to find someone to talk who will listen, when people look down on me and think they are more worthy than me, and when people call me names when they find out about my HIV status without giving me room to express myself.

You wonder where you would have gone to, but who could know? I'm so glad that it did work out and I've got to live my life in this bubble called HIV. I'm very open with my status, which gives me the opportunity to try to help others who need support. So, my life is very positive now – in both ways. I'm in a happy place.

Learning to protect myself through supportive connections

During my HIV journey, I have met some incredible people who have inspired me in so many ways. In all the charities I have volunteered and worked for, I have met so many people from all different walks of life and I I've learnt so many things from each one of them. I'm still learning, of course, but it's been an eye-opening experience.

As a result of these relationships, I have learnt to protect myself and I have to protect others, with regards to my health and safer sex by using condoms. I have also learnt the value of accepting things as they are and that you cannot control things.

Achievements and contributions within the HIV sector

- In December 2021, I received the Point of Light Award, which is recognised by the Prime Minister, who at the time was Boris Johnson.
- In 2019, I was awarded Islington Volunteer of The Year award for work with women living with HIV for my role in the HIV stigma campaigns.
- In 2019, I was also awarded the outstanding contribution NAZ project.
- In 2018, I was a poster girl for National Testing Week with the It Starts with Me campaign.
- In 2017, I was commissioned to make a Red Awareness brooch for Prince Harry and pinned it on him.
- I have also received a NOSCARS Sister Award for the work with Joyful Noise Choir NAZ Project.
- I was a central feature within an HIV awareness campaign. Having these posters displayed nationwide has supported people in the communities to step up and offer support and encouraged others to become activists and join the campaign for access and awareness of PrEP.

Life goes on.
My mind is positive.

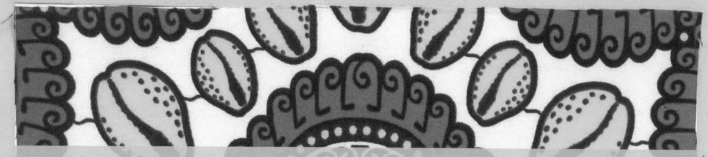

THE WEDDING AND WINTER THAT CHANGED MY LIFE: THE SILENCE OF HIV

Memory Sachikonye

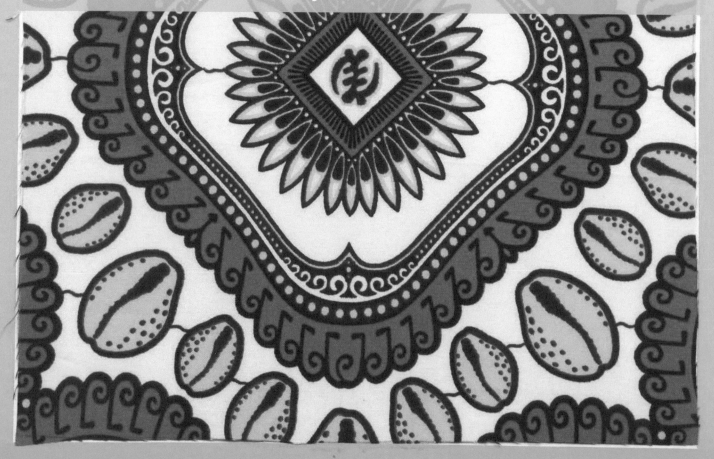

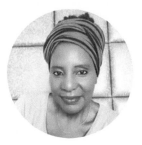

I was born in Zimbabwe and moved to the UK at the end of 2001. My mother was 19 when she had me. She was a single mother and had support from her father and sisters in raising me. Her own mother had passed away when she was nine years old, and as a result she had taken on the role of mother in her own family to mainly look after her own two young sisters and a brother. My mum went back to train as a teacher after she had me. The teacher's training college was at St Augustine's Penhalonga in the eastern highlands of Zimbabwe. This became the secondary school four of my siblings and my son would eventually attend.

I went to college and my first job was a receptionist for a publishing company. I had my son in 1987. I was a single mother but had my family's support.

In my working life I became a personal assistant for the founding directors of the company. My bosses had now formed a regional non-governmental organisation. The organisation did research and documented environment, democracy and women issues in the Southern Africa Development Community region. I was given the opportunity to study IT and managed the office computer network.

My story started after a shock HIV diagnosis in 2002 while on a three-week holiday to the UK. I didn't think then I would be here today. I had visited the UK several times before this visit. This visit was to a family wedding; my aunt was marrying her fifth husband on 21st December 2001. I arrived on 19th December. A few family members at the wedding remarked on how 'different' I looked. I had no idea what they were referring to.

The wedding went well, and we had a lovely Christmas. It snowed that year. I had a really bad cold and my aunt suggested I go for an HIV test. Twenty-four hours later, my whole life changed.

When I came to the UK, my son was 15 and midway through a boarding secondary school. I left my car parked at work. I gave my brother my bank card, so he could get some supplies for him when he went back to school. I left my home help at the house I was living in. My brothers and sister would be checking on her regularly. I didn't expect that I would not be returning back home after the wedding.

Back in Zimbabwe, in the late 1990s we lost five close family members to AIDS in a space of one year. We also lost a number of work colleagues. It was a difficult time; lots of people were dying yet no one spoke about the actual cause of death. It would say someone had died of malaria or diabetes – I guess the more acceptable causes of death.

There was nowhere to volunteer in Zimbabwe back then. Stigma was rife, with everyone trying to link sexual partners of the deceased so they could predict who would be the next person to fall sick and die. I had no reason to think I would be diagnosed with HIV later on. Information was also scarce and we relied on what the government issued.

Figuring out how things worked: what if I died before the doctor saw me?

After my diagnosis at St Ann's sexual health clinic in North London in January 2002, I had no idea how the NHS worked. I had been for the blood test 24 hours earlier. I can't remember anything that was said to me after being told I was HIV positive. My body and mind just shut down. All I remember is being told to wait for a letter to go to the hospital. I did not know where this hospital was. I just said OK and waited for the letter. My friend and relative asked about the test result; I told them, 'They said I am positive.'

I was lucky to be guided by my friend and a relative who was also living with HIV. We went to the North Middlesex Hospital on a bus. My relative was also accessing care there and told me that it would OK, but I did not believe her.

We got to reception and I was so welcomed by a nurse there. She knew my cousin by name. I was registered as a new patient and asked to get my bloods done. I was given an appointment to return in two weeks, the longest two weeks of my life! What if I died before the doctor could see me? Just having the diagnosis made me feel I was going back to Zimbabwe in a coffin. I had not seen anyone recover from AIDS, and everyone I had seen die had suffered miserably without any treatment.

After two weeks, I went back to the hospital, this time with my relative. As soon I got into reception, the receptionist greeted me by my first name. I smiled and responded nicely. In my mind, I thought my blood tests must so bad that the staff have been told to look for me. The AIDS stigma from Zimbabwe had followed me to the UK. I kept asking myself, how bad is my AIDS? It turned out that this receptionist/nurse had the memory of an elephant and knew everyone by name. She made the clinic a safe and pleasant place to visit. I then learnt that all the healthcare professionals working in HIV care were friendly and supportive to their patients.

I went in to see the doctor. He was very friendly and was looking at a computer screen at my results. He then told me I was to start treatment immediately – that is the only bit I also remember. I did not know what the medication would be. I come from a culture where you do not question health professionals. I did not ask a single question. All I understood was I had to take the tablets at the same time, every day, for life. My relative had told me what to expect. When we got home with my bags of meds, I took out the patient information sheet inside the tablet boxes to read. The purpose of the medication was to treat AIDS patients, it said. I knew this was real and embarked on my new life with medication.

The medication gave me terrible side effects, but I encouraged to persevere by my relative. One of the ARVs had to be taken at night, and it gave me horrible dreams and nightmares. On my next clinic visit two weeks later, I was hospitalised again.

A few weeks after starting treatment, I was very ill and was hospitalised for three weeks. I had a CD4 count of 6 and 65k viral load (which is high and a sign the virus was not under control); I had AIDS and suspected TB. I was also started on TB medication for six months. I was taking 18 tablets a day and had terrible side effects. I was quite ill and while in hospital I was also diagnosed with Adult Polycystic Kidney Disease. This is hereditary and runs in my father's side of the family.

The only thing I understood was that my immune system was responding to the medication. The TB medication has its own side effects, and I could not eat much. One of the tablets was huge and I struggled to swallow it. I asked if I could get it as a solution, but that solution tasted vile and the smell made me sick, but I still took it.

Navigating immigration and finding support

When I had stabilised and was out of hospital, I was referred to Positively Women for support. I walked into their offices on City Road and was taken into a room to be registered by a caseworker. The caseworker was a woman from Uganda. She looked glamorous with perfect make-up and a very warm smile. She introduced herself and told me she had been living with HIV for 17 years. After I picked up my jaw from the floor in disbelief, she explained what services were available from the organisation. She then took me to the open space where nearly 30 African women were talking and laughing. She had told me the room will be with other women living with HIV. I stood for a while wondering how these women could laugh when they had AIDS? Some were talking about sex. I had vowed never to have sex ever again. It was the cause of my current situation.

After my diagnosis, I got a lot of peer support from Positively Women, and got back my self-esteem and confidence. I was curious to understand more about my new-found disease. I was determined to free myself by being open about my status. I realised I could live well with the virus, besides other social challenges like dealing with immigration and the uncertainty of continuing with treatment if I were sent back to Zimbabwe.

I had learnt that I need to change my visa to stay. I was referred to a legal aid solicitor and my application as submitted before I overstayed. I then learnt that while the Home Office was deciding on my visa, I could not work or travel. Positively Women advertised for volunteers. I applied to volunteer with IT and a member of the editorial team for the bi-monthly women's magazine. This helped enhance my existing skills.

I have always been financially independent, and this was an adjustment I had to cope with. I am lucky to have close family members to stay with. I was eventually housed by my local social services and received £30 a week to buy food.

Volunteering for six-and-a-half years made me feel I was giving back to an organisation that helped. I also wanted to be a role model for other migrant women like me. A lot of us were anxiously waiting for a decision from the Home Office.

Three months into volunteering, I agreed to be on the cover of the Positively Women bi-monthly magazine. The magazine was circulated nationally. It was my way of telling my story and hopefully empowering women in my situation.

When I was out of hospital, I thought I could go home briefly to wrap up my work and collect my pension from my job of 14 years. The doctor smiled nicely and told me this would not be possible as I was still quite ill.

The highs and lows of living with HIV

The highs I believe are that I am alive today and getting the best care from the NHS. A lot of people in the world do not have this privilege. I was also empowered to be open about my HIV status, appeared as the cover girl on Positively Women magazine and Positive Nation – there was no going back. I was interviewed by CNN for World AIDS Day. This was broadcast on repeat throughout the day. I have been in newspaper and magazine articles with my picture and my name. My immigration issues took a long time to be dealt with, but that didn't stop me. My volunteering took me to meetings and involved me in other empowerment projects through Positively Women. I went to the House of Lords to tell my story as an asylum seeker living with HIV. I was determined to be heard.

I remember doing my first presentation at the first ever conference of people living with in Leicester where I told my story. I got very good reception from the 400 delegates. I still speak to small and large conferences and meetings.

One of the greatest highlights for me was being finally granted refugee status in 2008. I was reunited with my son in South Africa after 10 years.

Up until then I had lived in fear that the Home Office would refuse my application and send me back to Zimbabwe. My treatment in the UK was complex, none of which would be available in Zimbabwe at the time. It would be certain death if I were sent back home. I wanted to go home to be with my son, but knew I couldn't. Zimbabwe's economy was struggling then and still is.

Some of the lows of living with HIV have been the anxiety of an uncertain future in the UK. Depression, anxiety and isolation could have been easily become my friends. I volunteered and engaged with my local council, health providers and peers as a way of coping or staying sane.

Another low point for me was finding out that my son had known about my HIV status without me telling him, which was heart breaking. I had planned to find the right time to tell him after his A-levels, but unfortunately the internet was faster than me. He had no problem with my status, but was pissed off about the way he found out.

Living well with HIV, friends, family and my professional work

My family has always been very supportive. I told them about my diagnosis. My mother would call and text all the time. If I didn't respond to a text quick enough, she would worry. I cannot imagine what she must have felt being more than 10,000 miles away. I did all I could to reassure her I was in good hands. My siblings and extended family are still my biggest cheerleaders. They fully support everything I do.

I am that person in family WhatsApp groups who shares information about HIV. I have been talking about U=U lately. This is hoping to help fight stigma and also empower those silent voices. I am also on Zimbabwean social media groups and always comment and share correct, up-to-date HIV information.

I have met and made friends for life in HIV. I have attended various support groups in the early years. I learnt and shared a lot with my HIV peers. At some point, I outgrew the support groups. I had three close friends from Positively Women (Angelina, Rebecca and Charity). The other friend (Winnie) I had known from AHPN. We got together one evening and decided we would support each other at a different level. Our home countries are Zimbabwe, Zambia, Uganda and Kenya. We chose the name ZZUK Africa United and use the acronym ZZUK. Years later, that sisterhood had achieved a lot, from making and selling Africa-inspired goods to writing this book. We socialise and have great respect for each other. I am still friends with other women I met at Positively Women.

Being open about my HIV status has made me approachable to people who want to share their status with me. I have supported family members; besides their healthcare professionals, I am the only other person they have shared their story with. These are people who are not ready to be seen. They ask for advancements in treatment, they want to know when the HIV cure is coming. Each time I go on a trip, I have one friend who will ring me and say, 'What new things do they have for us?'

My HIV consultant, who retired in 2022, was also a good friend. As chair of the patient forum, my clinic visit was in three parts – medical, clinic business and social. He was one doctor who was always late with appointments. You knew you would wait over an hour after your appointment time. All patients understood that he was thorough with all his patients and did not mind waiting. There is an important bond that HIV doctors develop with their patients. I used to say my doctor has been in my life for 20 years, which is the longest relationship I have had with one man. He is known as my HIV husband; he knows, too.

My work involves working with HIV doctors, researchers and other professionals. This has empowered me as a patient. I am the patient voice on study management groups with high-ranking professionals. I feel listened to and respected. I am named as an author in publications.

Some of the things that I have learnt along the way are that we are all patient leaders. The NHS sets up engagement structures without being too bothered about building the capacity of those involved. As patient leaders, we often deal with professionals in most cases unaided. Patient engagement must take place early and should not be seen as an add-on. It needs to take place in time for the results to be able to influence the final result.

Patients must be allowed a genuine opportunity to make a difference, not paid lip service!

We should engage the younger generation to keep the passion alive, while being professional, and pass this on to future patient leaders.

Over the years my contributions to HIV activism have been:

- Chair of the HIV Patient Forum at North Middlesex Hospital.
- Contributing to HIV research as a patient rep on various HIV studies, the longest being the POPPY study on HIV and ageing.
- UK-CAB co-ordinator, which helps ensure patient voices are heard and represented on clinical study committees and advisory board. We have patient reps on the BHIVA and NHIVNA executive committees.
- Service user rep for the HIV Strategic Forum in Enfield and Haringey through my HIV clinic.
- Service user rep for the Physical Disabilities Board in Enfield to ensure HIV stayed on their agenda.

- Worked with Enfield Social Services, which was awarded Beacon status for services to disabled adults in 2008.
- Coordinated UMOJA, a mixed HIV service for Afro-Caribbean people living in Enfield – most of us also had immigration and social issues.

My greatest achievement was supporting a young woman from Zimbabwe more than 10 years ago. She was referred to me by my brother, who is a medical doctor. His brief to me was to help her accept her HIV status. We started chatting on WhatsApp. Her biggest concern was about having children. She already had one son before her diagnosis. I explained the importance of staying on her ARVs and also speak to her doctor in case she needed to change her meds before conceiving. We chatted regularly about general health and other things.

A year later, I got a message with a picture of a baby boy. She just said, 'Here is your grandson. Thank you for all the support.' I was so happy for her. She had followed all the advice and her son was healthy. Our relationship grew stronger, and another year later she had a second son. I met up with her on my first visit to Zimbabwe in 2017. It was the best feeling ever! We still chat regularly. They boys are growing up nice and are all in school.

You are bigger than HIV. Do not let the virus shape who you are.

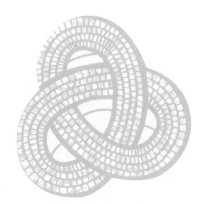

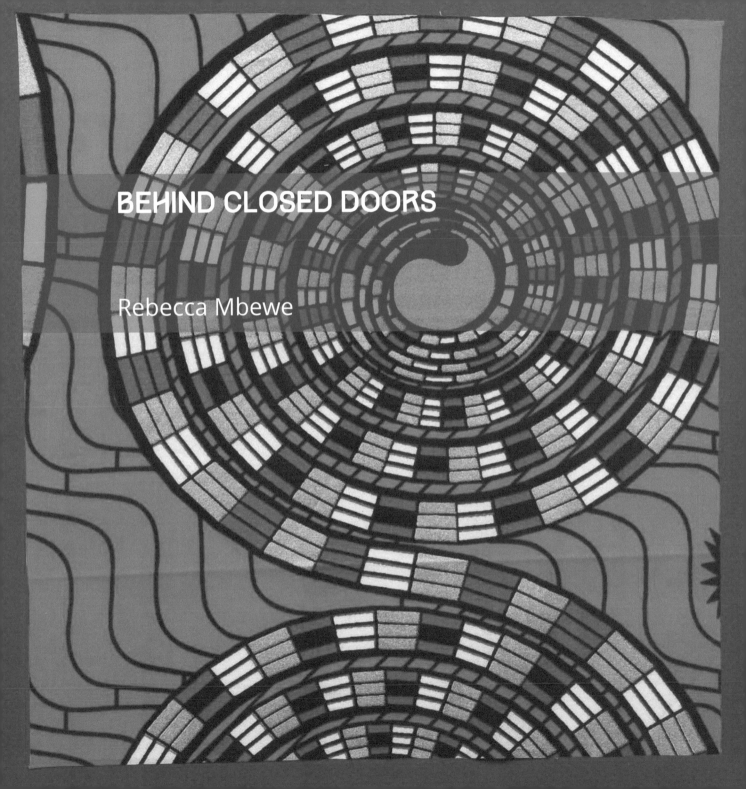

BEHIND CLOSED DOORS

Rebecca Mbewe

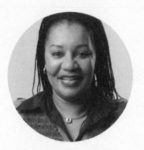

My life journey begins in the small town of Ndola in Zambia, a beautiful landlocked country in sub-Saharan Africa. I was born in January 1968 and am the eldest of four children – though my two younger brothers have since passed away. My mother was one of those women with many talents. She could bake, knit, sew, crochet and a whole lot of other things – you name it, she could do it. Because of this she was always busy either helping out with school fetes or helping organising Rotarian functions. As a South African woman who migrated to Zambia, she was a bit of an outlier. She smoked and drank and was never afraid to speak her mind. Somehow, she managed to do all of those things with the grace and poise of a lady. My mother ran a nursery school where we often helped out during school holidays. It was really popular and considered to have very high standards, which meant the waiting list would sometimes be up to a year.

My father was the typical Black African man of those times. He was the complete opposite of my mother, who was quite petite and fair in complexion. My father was tall, very dark and handsome. He was very principled and quite stern. I only ever saw him laugh in the company of his friends. I recall him being able to speak five languages, so you can imagine his level of expectation for us. He was an accountant by profession, which meant of course he was very savvy with numbers. He often got very frustrated helping us with our maths homework because we couldn't think as quickly as he could. I remember him telling me not to 'think like a chicken' – to this day I am not quite sure what he meant, perhaps implying I had a small brain. I will never know.

Even though my father was the disciplinarian of our family, as was the case with most fathers of that generation, he did have a soft side, the side that would whisper to the fruit trees in the orchard. Through his patience, he grew plums and other fruit that would not normally bear in warm weather. He was very proud of this. It was from him that I learnt what grafting was. He also reared chickens – as many as 4,000 at one point! We were expected to help out with feeding the chickens. This is where I learnt to slaughter and dress chickens.

I remember my childhood as quite happy with lots of fun memories. We had a very sheltered upbringing and spent most, if not all of our childhood not venturing far off from our homes. Our lives evolved around going to school, church and back home again. Every Christmas, we would go to family gatherings and my parents would often have a New Year party that was the go-to event of the year and was always the talk of the town. I realise now that I am grown that it was probably because there was an abundance of alcohol and food. People arrived all glammed up and didn't leave until the very early hours of the next day!

We had many pets. Other than the usual dogs, we had rabbits, guinea pigs and at one point a tortoise that was large enough for us to ride. We also had what we thought was a monkey until a friend of my dad's friend pointed out it was a young baboon that as an adult could become aggressive and not particularly good to have around young girls. That was the end of Charlie, who was taken to the local zoo the very next weekend. That was a great excuse to go to the zoo more regularly though.

I went to Kansenji Primary School for the first five years of my education and then transferred to the Dominican Convent School for Girls. At the time I joined it had both primary and secondary facilities, so I completed my primary education there and went on to attend the first three years of my secondary education there as well. I then transferred to a newly opened Church of England Secondary School for my final secondary years of Form 4 and 5.

I was active and got involved in all the sporting activities. We did not have much choice because it was a compulsory part of the curriculum, but I actually enjoyed any sporting activity. I joined everything but netball, maybe because I was overshadowed by the girls much taller than me. I did partake in hockey, running, high jump, long jump, discus and javelin. Swimming was my favourite, but I also loved drama with equal passion. I learnt to swim from a very early age, so was very good by the time I went to secondary school. I joined the cadets and did very well – I attained the level of Staff Sergeant by the time it was stopped as an extracurricular school activity. Looking back, it was a shame that the government chose to stop the cadets because they considered the training too harsh for young children. However, I enjoyed my time there and learnt so much. All this activity fitted very well with my tomboy character. I absolutely loved it! It was not encouraged by my father, though, because he thought drama, singing, dancing and anything that was not academic was a total waste of time.

Basically, my childhood was great until I learnt at the age of 15 that the man who had raised me was not my biological father, causing me much confusion. All this was to play out over the coming years. I learnt that my biological father was a pilot who lived in Lusaka, the capital of Zambia. I learnt that he was married and had two boys. I was told there was another girl older than myself, so there were two of us from before he was married.

The events of history shaping the future

The year 1985 was a life-changing year for me. I was in my final year of secondary school with lots of plans to study pharmacology. As a family we were also going through quite a few big changes – we moved house from a much larger house, one where we had invested a lot of time, blood, sweat and tears. It was a home we built from the ground up – everything from the grass, the plants and the trees to my mum's nursery school, the chicken runs and orchard, so it was heart-breaking to have to move. We moved to a company house because my father had bought a smallholding and had plans to develop the exact same outlay as the house that we moved from but as life would have it, the universe had other plans. Not long after we moved to the new area, my youngest brother was born and given there was 13 years' difference between him and my brother before him, we were also just getting used to the youngest addition to our family. It was a complicated birth that Mum never really recovered from. She died in July 1985, and this left a great big hole in all of our lives. Being the oldest, I had to grow up literally overnight, both mentally and practically. I became a carer for my siblings and took to looking after my four-month-old brother during the night and would have to get up the next day to rush to school. During the day I relied on my other brother, as he was waiting on his exam results to go into secondary school, and happened to have a longer break off school. I would rush home at 3pm to prepare dinner and take over looking after the baby. My grades were badly affected and consequently, my final GSE O-level result was poor. This went on for a whole year until a close friend of my mother's gave me the best advice ever.

She sat me down and said, 'Rebecca, I know right now you think the best way of looking after your siblings is through the way you are doing now. But I promise you, the best you can do for them is returning to education, bettering yourself and making sure you are established enough to support them.'

That was the most honest advice I had been given at the time. I started to think about how I could further my education with the low grades I had achieved. In Zambia, to get anywhere you either had to know someone or have proof of excellent grades, neither of which I had. Anyway, a year later my biological father passed away and I went to his funeral, where I got to meet new family members. I acquired new family members overnight – aunts, uncles, siblings, my grandmother and grandfather from my father's side. I also met eight of my other siblings. Other than the one who was older than me, all the others were from after his marriage. You can imagine how eventful the funeral was!

It was at the funeral that my aunt – my father's sister – offered to pay for me to go to secretarial college. Much to my non-biological father's anger and disappointment, I enrolled in the college, got accepted and went off to secretarial college for the next 18 months. I completed the course with flying colours and got a job initially with an import and export company and later one of the biggest banks in the country. It was through my first job that I met the man I eventually married and who was to become the father of my two children.

Love, marriage, new arrivals and the start of a new UK chapter

We got married in December 1990, four months after the birth of our first son. After a few years, my husband had the opportunity to further his career and left to study in England. He travelled in 1994 and we joined in September of the following year. Coming to England was a complete culture shock. Getting terribly sunburnt was the first surprising experience and long days and nights was the other! We learnt about it, but never quite imagined it in the way that I saw it.

Apart from my husband and sister-in-law, I knew no one. There was a lot to learn in terms of navigating the system; life in general was very fast paced, unlike my home country. I arrived to find my husband had not been able to study very much because he was constantly ill. I did what I know best and very quickly adapted to taking care of my poorly husband and young child. As his health was getting progressively worse, it was recommended by our GP that we took an HIV test. With no real understanding of what that meant, we arrived at the Royal Free Hospital, where we undertook the tests and were advised that we would be contacted after two weeks.

I was quite naive and didn't realise what having an HIV positive diagnosis meant. I therefore went along with life as normal and in hindsight can see that I didn't really have the same anxieties as that of my husband. I was more preoccupied with the day-to-day activities in our lives. We eventually were asked to come back to the hospital, where we were probably counselled prior to being given the results – my memory of that day is vague. All I remember is asking the doctor if it was possible to check my son as I had breast fed him. Fortunately, my son was negative, which was a huge relief, even though I couldn't have told you why at the time. It just felt that way given people's reactions and responses around me. The staff and care was amazing. I still access care from the same centre.

Living a double life

Life became more difficult, having to manage my husband's hospital admissions, a full-time job, looking after my child, sorting out accommodation and immigration matters, as well as increasing domestic violence. My husband constantly blamed me for 'bringing this thing into our home'! My saving grace was that I was referred to peer support almost immediately after my diagnosis and was able to access support through the weekly groups they held at Positively Women. It was the only space I felt I could have any peace, even if only for a few hours.

I led a double life – as a woman living with HIV in an unhappy marriage and as a professional woman working in a highly prestigious law firm. This continued for many years. I got pregnant in 1999 with my second son, who was born HIV free thanks to the various interventions at the time. As per the guidelines at the time, I had a planned caesarean birth, did not breastfeed and went on to treatment for the duration of the pregnancy, even though I did not require it for myself. I felt blessed that I did not need to start treatment straight away as I was in fairly good health, and having supported my husband through his treatment regime it was the one thing I was most afraid of. I often imagined how I would cope having to take so many medications and having to manage them with their different requirements. Some needed to be taken with food, others without, and it was quite a job just managing the medication.

My husband's health did not improve, and he eventually died in 2002. I was left to bring up two young boys in a foreign country and manage my own health, all whilst maintaining a full-time job and dealing with all the other issues of being a migrant. Fortunately, my peer support organisation was extremely supportive and provided both emotional and practical support when we needed it.

With the demise of my husband, my responsibilities of being a carer were of course now redundant and therefore freed up a bit more time, which I dedicated to becoming a bit more involved in the organisation where I was accessing support. I initially started by being a service user representative and began contributing to the organisation's monthly magazine. I wrote articles and was part of the editorial team.

All the while, I was still leading this double life. I had done very well in my professional life, settling into a legal PA role for a media law firm in the city. Shortly after my husband's death, I fell very ill and could not continue working for this company. They were extremely helpful in trying to keep me on the payroll as long as they could, paying for alternative therapies that I would otherwise not have been able to afford. My boss at the time was the first person I told about my circumstances – that my husband was dying in hospital and I was living with HIV. I received such a positive response; my boss was more worried about me resigning! We eventually reached a mutual agreement, that I would resign as they could no longer keep me on the payroll. I took the opportunity to relocate outside London where we lived for 18 months. After I had fully recovered, I started working in Kettering, but life was not sustainable as the salaries were very low.

Another chance that helped shape my life

We returned to London, where I managed to get work in another law firm where I stayed for another couple of years before I decided to return to full-time study. I enrolled on a BSc Psychology with Counselling Theory at a University in West London and achieved second class honours. This was something I was very proud of because it felt like I had been given another chance to redeem my poor GCE grades. And I did this all whilst raising a family and running a home – all I can say is respect to adult learning!!! Whilst I was studying, I applied to volunteer with Positively Women as it was known at the time, at its women's group in Hammersmith. When the role of caseworker came up, I applied and got the job. It was an amazing experience and one that would shape the next phase of my life. I learnt a huge amount and gained a lot of experience of working not only on different cases, but also from working with different professionals and organisations. I remained in the role for seven years and throughout became more and more involved in support, mentoring and speaking engagements.

Over the years, I have worked in various organisations in different capacities, such as in prevention and testing and even in operations. I have sat on several advisory groups and been a trustee on others. I have participated in research and contributed to scholarly articles, all hugely beneficial to my growth and professional development in the field of HIV. I went on to study for my MBA in Healthcare and graduated in 2018. Even though I stepped away from the HIV sector for a couple of years, I was always involved in some way or another. I continued to work with the 4M Mentor Mother's Network CIC, an organisation focused on supporting women living with HIV going through the perinatal journey. It has developed from simply being a project to becoming its own entity and continues to grow from strength to strength.

At the time of writing this, I am co-leading the GROWS Project, a programme for Women over 40 ageing with HIV. I continue to sit on the British HIV Association (BHIVA) Audit Standards Subcommittee, and I am a proud UK Community Advisory Board (UK-CAB) member.

There are many times, I have felt proud of my achievements, but if I were to pick a few it would include being one of the speakers at the launch of the Fast Track Cities Initiative alongside London Mayor Sadiq Khan and great allies such as Professor Jane Anderson and Professor Kevin Fenton. My other most memorable moment is meeting Winnie Byanyima, Executive Director of UNAIDS at an event organised by STOPAIDS.

Acquiring more than a formal education

There have certainly been many lows of my journey as well as many highs. I have heard from many what a positive impact my support has had on their lives, but what they do not know is that each and every encounter I have had has impacted me and made me more determined to continue to do the work I do, to speak on behalf of those that are unable to do so for themselves. Working within HIV has taught me way more than any formal education could have. I have become more understanding and accepting of differences, more patient and knowledgeable of the differences we have and the challenges we encounter as human beings regardless of our journey or background. It has been a great honour to meet the people I have met in my life and will continue to meet.

Looking back, even though I felt completely helpless at times, I would say to my younger self have faith in your own strength and resilience, as this is what will carry you through and you will be all right. Whilst I feel achieving a higher level of education has been quite rewarding, given the challenges along the way, the most important achievements for me are those that have involved other people living with HIV. There is nothing more valuable than watching someone I had the privilege of meeting in their most vulnerable circumstance thriving because of that interaction. That is a wonderful achievement and the most important one for me.

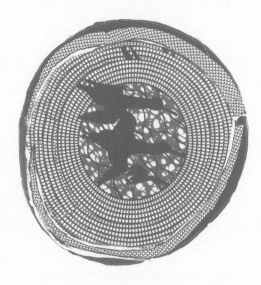

Have faith in your own strength and resilience, as it will carry you through.

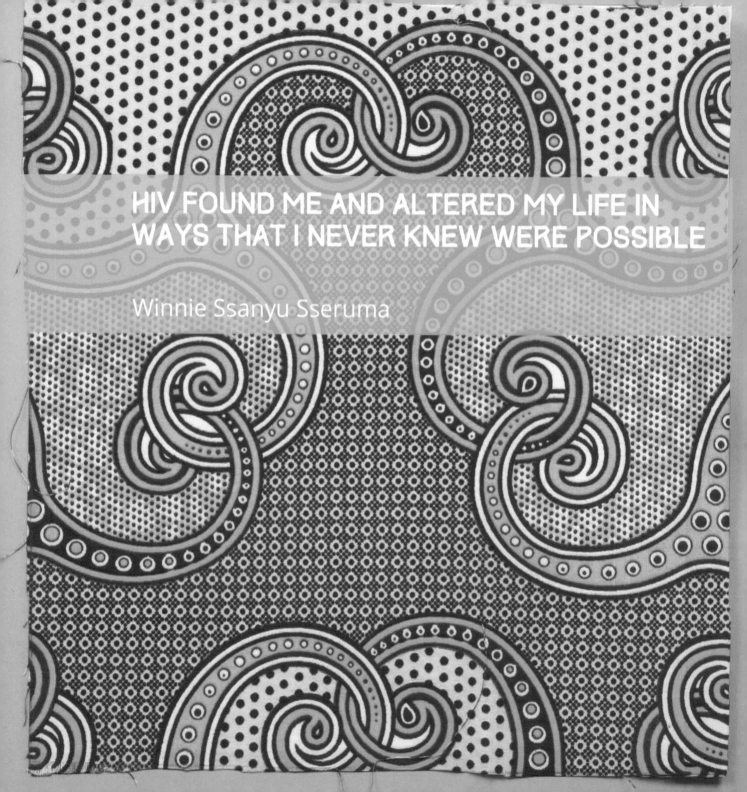

HIV FOUND ME AND ALTERED MY LIFE IN WAYS THAT I NEVER KNEW WERE POSSIBLE

Winnie Ssanyu Sseruma

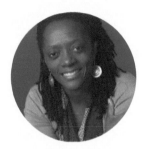

grew up in Uganda, my ancestral home, but I was born in Sheffield, UK. Both of my parents were teachers, they valued education and made sure that my four siblings and I were able to get into what were some of the best schools in Uganda, at the time.

My formative years were spent in faith-based boarding schools, mostly Catholic and one Islamic school. I felt very much that due to attending boarding schools until about the age of 16, I was cocooned, naive about a lot of things and lived in a bubble. While boarding schools in the UK are seen as places where rich people take their children to get the best education money can buy, in many places in Africa it is very different. Parents took and continue to take their children to boarding schools for mostly practical reasons. Boarding schools are perceived to offer the best education, there are fewer distractions for children, and children are well looked after. These schools are convenient for parents who work and don't have time to ferry their children to school every day. Perhaps it even works out cheaper. Daily travel on what is considered public transport in many African countries can be costly, insecure and inconsistent, among many other things. Anyway, these are just some thoughts, not an exhaustive list. The point is, in Africa boarding schools are not for the children of the elite.

I felt that growing up in Uganda, my family life was good most of the time. Our family was close, we had most of what we needed and as a child I felt loved. But national governments' politics have always been punctuated by political skirmishes, coups and full-blown wars. There were times when I was terrified, saw stuff no child or adult should see or experience, but I thought that it was all part of life – normal.

After my A-levels in 1981, I got a scholarship and went to study at the University of Saint Mary, in Kansas, USA. While it was a relief to leave Uganda (due to political turmoil, lack of further education opportunities or work prospects), I worried about my family and missed them all the time. Although Saint Mary University felt like just another boarding school to me, the cultural shock was off the scale. As a Black African, I was in the minority at the school. There was so much to learn, and this is where I really came face to face with the issue of race and what it means to be black in the USA.

I graduated with a BA in Sociology in 1985, but was unable to return to Uganda, because the country was a war zone. In 1987, I went back briefly, mostly because I was so homesick. It was a relief to see my whole family, but it was a difficult time. The people and the country were just starting to recover from war.

I returned to the USA in mid-1988 to build on my Sociology degree and to get some practical skills. To be honest, even as I continued my studies I wasn't sure what my end goal was in terms of a career. I felt I was just going through the motions of what I thought growing up was supposed to be.

HIV found me and altered my life, in ways that I never knew were possible

I was diagnosed with HIV in 1988 at 27 years of age, eight years before I moved to the UK. I was diagnosed through what I would compare to an internship programme, part of an interview process where I was required to take various blood tests because I was going to be interacting with patients. Testing positive for HIV was a shock, to say the least. It completely changed the direction of my life.

In the 1980s, there was no living with HIV, just dying from it in the most horrendous of ways. It really was the stuff of nightmares. Two weeks after my diagnosis, I was offered the first single HIV treatment, which at the time was on the market in the USA mostly for emergency use. AZT was supposed to prolong the lives of people who had HIV at the time. Gay men, many fighting for their lives, forced the US government to approve it quickly, in order to save lives. While bringing AZT on the market may have seemed like a hopeful sign, many people didn't survive the toxicity of the drug. The side effects were terrible and experienced differently by individuals. I experienced nausea, loss of appetite, loss of weight, ashy skin, darkened fingernails and toenails and much more. To this day, I am still not sure how I survived it.

As scientists and doctors learnt more about HIV and how to treat it, not to mention the pressure from mainly gay activists at the time, more HIV drugs were introduced, but they remained really toxic. In the following years, I was started on dual therapy AZT and DDI, but I was struggling physically, especially with side effects. Emotionally and mentally, I was not well either. I had not shared my HIV status with anyone outside of my health clinic.

In the early 1990s after losing both my parents to different forms of cancer and a younger brother to HIV-related TB, I also began to lose the will to live. In 1994, I returned to Uganda with a focus on dying. Once my medication ran out, I was ravaged by opportunistic infections including TB, pneumonia and diarrhoea. However, because I knew what was ailing me, and with the financial ability to access private care and support from my sister, I survived. In 1996, I travelled to the UK as part of my convalescing for a two-week vacation with some of my siblings, a niece and a nephew. I had no intention of residing in the UK, even though it is my birthplace. I really didn't want to start a new life. I still wanted what I thought was my imminent death to happen in Uganda. Morbid, I know. Mentally, I was in a really bad space.

What was different in 1996 was that highly active anti-retroviral treatment (HAART) was available in the UK and was starting to change the HIV landscape. HAART was so effective, its impact on people living with HIV was referred to in biblical terms as the Lazarus effect.

Out of boredom and not having planned much to do, during my vacation I attended an HIV support group for the first time since my diagnosis. It was sold to me as a meeting to talk and meet people. I attended the group at Body and Soul, an HIV support organisation that had a weekly group for heterosexual women and men living with HIV, and a space for both young people and children. When I attended the support group, mostly African women stood up and talked about how they nearly died and then felt better again through accessing treatment, social and emotional support. With HIV treatment, they were once again feeling alive, even though many had felt very poorly. Their lives had turned around in a few days of starting the lifesaving treatments.

When I left that support group that day, my thinking had already started to shift from focusing on dying to thinking that perhaps a small window of hope had just opened. I thought that if the brave women I had seen and heard speak, were able to turn their lives around, what was stopping me? I went back to the hospital a few days later, asked to be started on HIV treatment and embarked on a new life in the UK. It was not easy, but I have never looked back. That was the start of my HIV activism.

There was no living with HIV, just dying from it

My life dramatically changed when I received my HIV diagnosis. However, while I initially thought that I was doomed to a premature death, every day since continues to surprise me in many different ways.

On much reflection, the decade from 1990 to 2000 was the worst of times but it was also so important on my HIV journey. Let me explain. At the beginning of the 1990s both my parents died within two years of each other, and I lost one of my younger brothers. That was half my family gone. The stress of dealing with the deaths of three family members so close together, as well as dealing with what I thought was my impending death, was unbearable at times. Although I was never clinically diagnosed with depression, I certainly felt like I was in a very bad place mentally.

The series of events led me to return to Uganda in 1994 to wait out what I thought would be my last days on earth. For most of the two years I was in Uganda, I was nursing one opportunistic infection after another, once my HIV treatment run out. I spent a lot of time on my own with my drear thoughts. I suppose some of my relatives were concerned, but none of them felt they could to talk me about my HIV. No one wanted to talk about it then; very few still do.

When I arrived in the UK in 1996 and started accessing emotional and social support, as well as effective HIV treatment, my life completely turned around 180 degrees. I completely recovered from my previous opportunistic infections, I got my energy back, I started sharing my lived experience of HIV and I built a whole new life in the UK. I went from desperately not wanting to live to living with intent. It was a remarkable transformation.

As I have described, it wasn't one specific thing that made life terrible at the beginning of the 1990s and equally it wasn't just a single issue that helped me turn my life around. My HIV journey continues. I feel that I continue to survive through a series of coincidences, opportunities, being in the right place at the right time, believing in and embracing medical science, networking, connections and always tapping into my inner strength to get through each day.

Building meaningful relationships: the HIV community I joined

Relationships matter and are fundamental to building communities. I have met numerous people on my continuing HIV journey and built some very unlikely relationships. I strongly feel there is something very special about the HIV community, not just at a national but also at global level.

The HIV community I am referring to and highlighting here, is one that I would not have wanted to be associated with. In fact, I remember at one point standing up and saying I didn't feel like being part of it. But what is it they say again? You live and learn! In this particular instance, I am happy to have lived long enough to be part of the HIV community – benefiting from it as well as contributing.

HIV remains one of the most stigmatised conditions, and HIV-related stigma is one of the biggest challenges we continue to struggle to eliminate. What many people who are not associated with HIV do not realise is that stigma kills. HIV-related stigma keeps people from accessing the support and services they need, such as HIV testing, knowledge on how to protect themselves, HIV treatment, social support and so much more. People have died and continue to die because they can't bear to talk to anyone about their positive HIV status, even in this era where treatment has enabled us to live well and stopped the transmission of HIV.

When I was first diagnosed, like many other people living with HIV, I prepared for a horrific death, not a long life. Announcing that you were living with HIV was inviting ostracisation, violence, social exclusion and in some instances death. Why would you then associate yourself with anything that could link you to HIV?

Nevertheless, many people found themselves in very difficult circumstances ostracised by those that they cared about the most, especially when HIV intersected with any number of cultural, religious and social norms. People living with HIV were forced to come together to fight to survive.

While we had common goals to work towards as an HIV community, it was never easy. Many of us had never worked together and some groups were fearful of others. But reversing the injustices that many of us were facing and with HIV as the most common theme – white gay men, Black Africans, migrants, commercial sex workers, haemophiliacs, people who use drugs, black gay men, lesbians and so many other groups came together at small and big HIV meetings in the UK and internationally, and we all advocated together. I had never attended so many meetings on one subject in my life and I had a steep learning curve to navigate, to understand not only the cross-cutting issues, but also who was who in terms of policy-makers, government officials and what we were supposed to be asking for. It was a crash course in learning to do advocacy, campaigning, public speaking, movement building, the science of HIV treatments and so much more, all rolled into one. It was hard, confusing at times and exhausting, but it was also engaging, educational and very addictive.

Over the last quarter of a century, relationships have been built ranging from work relationships to strong friendships. An amazing HIV community, which I am very proud to be part of, has been built, involving not only those of us living with HIV, but also allies such as HIV physicians, policy-makers, CEOs of various organisations/businesses, pharmaceutical company representatives, members of parliament, church leaders, celebrities and so many more. The HIV community includes incredible individuals who continue to make history, a family that supports so many of us on our HIV journeys.

You live and you learn: the achievements that I am proud of

As ironic as it sounds, I feel that living with HIV gave me a purpose to strive and to live for. Many naive and uninformed people continue to believe that living with HIV is one of the worst things that can happen to you. I can say that, like with everything in life, it depends on who you talk to. Different people have different experiences.

I have now been living with HIV for more than half my life. I felt I had to work with the cards I was dealt. It was either that or die. I nearly did at one point. What I could not have planned for or expected was a productive and fulfilling life after my diagnosis. It is a joy to be alive and maturing with HIV at 61 years of age.

It wasn't until I settled in the UK in 1996 that I started to talk about my lived experience of HIV. I did so because I felt supported emotionally and health-wise. I also felt well enough to share my story to encourage others to access services they need. I thought that I would share my story a couple of times and that would be it. Little did I know that I was at the beginning of my HIV activism. Talking and writing about my HIV diagnosis, the lows, the ultra-lows and how I lived long enough to access effective antiretroviral therapy was liberating. I have met people who have told me that I touched their lives in ways I didn't expect. This put me on a trajectory to reclaim my life in ways I didn't think were possible.

There are many things I am proud to have done and to be involved with, but I can only write about very few in this book. I am proud of the work that I did when I was supported by HIV i-Base, to train as an HIV treatment advocate. The HIV treatment literacy programme and other support work I did as an employee of this organisation continues to play an important role in my life. Understanding the medical science on how HIV treatments work, not only helped me to become an expert patient in my health, but also enabled me to empower others to improve their treatment literacy. Treatment literacy opened up a whole new world for me, a skill that I continue to build on and adapt to other health conditions.

I also worked for Christian Aid UK for almost a decade, and part of my initial role was training all staff in the UK and internationally on HIV. At one point, HIV awareness training was one of the compulsory trainings every new staff member had to attend. I constantly reviewed the training and at some point added a section on HIV treatments, the various classes of treatments, how they work to suppress the HIV virus and the advocacy around access to treatment for all. In their anonymous evaluations at the end of each training, most of those attending indicated that the section of HIV treatments was most interesting and informative. In addition to the pride I felt about the HIV training, many staff members, privately told me that I helped change their attitudes around HIV for the better, because of the way I carried myself at work and how I lived openly with my HIV status.

When I left Christian Aid, I decided to do freelance consultancy work, building on my HIV work, international development skills and networks. I have had great opportunities to facilitating trainings with people living with HIV, participate and facilitate community research, programme evaluations and to be part of discussions that have initiated policy change. By far one of the highlights of my working life has been my work as a Field Representative for The Stephen Lewis Foundation, which is based in Toronto, Canada. Through this work, I monitor and assess community health and social enterprise initiatives in 15 countries across Africa whose work is anchored in working on HIV and AIDS. Travelling through parts of Africa I never dreamt of travelling to and talking to women living with HIV, young people, grandmothers, the LGBTQI communities being supported by local community based organisations and the impact that has had on their lives, have been some of the most fulfilling and rewarding experiences. It is the best education, I never had about my beloved continent.

In the UK, I come across many people who ask me if people's lives are changing for the better in Africa, especially where HIV is concerned. I would like to say emphatically that yes, they are, because I have heard many testimonies supporting all sorts of transformations. This is not to say that challenges don't exist, they do. There is a need to rethink how those challenges can be better addressed to have a more sustainable impact. Additionally, we all need to get better at telling a different and positive (no pun intended) story about Africa, rather than the still stereotypical one of those people who can't help themselves.

Create your own family

I have learnt so much through living with HIV and still learning. One of the most important lessons is being kind to myself no matter what else is going on. Self-care is so important. One of the best things I ever did for myself was accessing one-to-one counselling to deal with issues I was struggling to work through and or to come to terms with. I can't recommend counselling enough to properly and effectively deal with challenging issues

Surround yourself with a small support network of friends who you can share ideas with, have fun with and rely on to have your back and you, theirs. Families come in all shapes and sizes; create your own that serves your evolving needs.

Practise empathy and learn to work in partnership with others. Working with others, especially when you have very little in common can sometimes be challenging. Throughout my years of HIV activism, I have attended numerous meetings, round-table discussions and conferences. In most of these spaces, different points of views were represented. Sometimes there were a lot of disagreements, tensions ran high, and sometimes the anger that people felt was overwhelming and got the better of them. What I found useful was listening and learning about what I knew little or nothing about. It has been an education watching how ideas and discussions come together, turn into campaign asks, to bring people together once again for the cause.

Live.
Listen.
Learn.
Love.
Laugh.
Life is really
what you
make it.

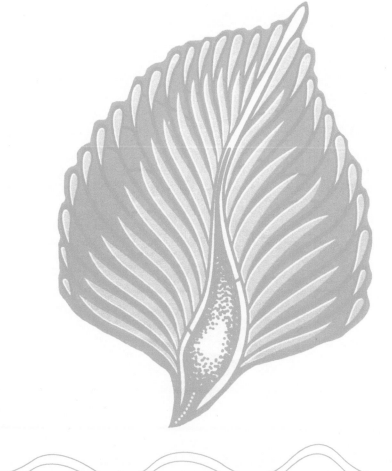

IF YOU NEED ME

If you need me, I will be
the family you choose.
If you need me, tell me.
Talk to me.
I may not have all the answers,
but I am ready to listen.
If you need me, I will be
your sounding-board.
Don't hesitate to call!
Sharing is caring after all.
If you need me, I'll be there.
Any time of the day,
morning noon or night.
Just pick up the phone and WhatsApp me.
(My phone is permanently on silent!)

If you need me, I will give you

cuddles and happiness,

hold your hand and be there for you.

I will not judge you for who you are.

You will always be my friend.

If you need me,

I'll be there. (Like that very famous Diana Ross song!)

I'll be there. I'll be there.

Group poem

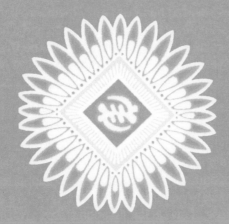

EXPERIENCES OF PEOPLE LIVING WITH HIV

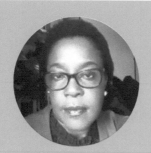

A CUP OF TEA AND A DIAGNOSIS OF HIV: RESPONDING TO MY HIV DIAGNOSIS

Adela Senkubuge

grew up in Uganda and I'm the last of seven children. I'm in my late 50s and I'm a mother of an adult son, who is a lawyer. I have many nephews and nieces. I say I have many children. Before I was diagnosed, I was working in print media, with a government in Uganda. I also had a small business doing flower arrangements for different events, so I had a side income. I started a group to help women become financially independent in my village.

In 2002, I moved to the UK. I was losing weight, but I didn't know why. After some time, I had a health check where they also checked for HIV. I was asked to come back after two weeks. I was given a cup of tea, the usual British way of doing things. Then I was told that I was living with HIV. I remember keeping quiet. Oh, my God! I had three thoughts, which I still remember very clearly. First, can I survive? Is there a miracle for me to survive HIV? At the time HIV was killing people. I had lost my friends; I had lost family members back home. I knew what it looked like because I had seen people living with HIV who had died. Second, I thought about my son. How was he going to grow up without me? The third thought that stuck with me was, if I live for one year, if I live for three months, if I live for ten years, this virus will never leave me.

Finding a new family

When I was referred to a UK charity, near to where I lived at the time, I didn't know there was such support for people living with HIV. I didn't know that people could meet, talk about their experiences, make friends, network and learn. This organisation supported me from the beginning. The support involved how to adhere to treatment, take care of myself and follow a healthy diet. However, because of my UK immigration status, I wasn't sure how I was going to stay and receive this treatment and care. I was reassured to learn that HIV treatment is free in the UK. I started volunteering in the HIV sector. I wanted to share my experience and support others through their journey.

There were so many tablets that I had to take. I still tell people that when you're coming from countries where treatment is not readily available, all you want is treatment. I didn't care whether there were six tablets or twenty – if they were going to save my life I would take as many as was needed. I never had any problems adhering to the tablets because I knew wholeheartedly my life depended on it. However, after six months on these tablets, I developed stomach problems. It was terrible and my consultant changed it to another combination, which helped a lot.

When I moved to Manchester, I remember I was given an envelope before I left London with information about the hospitals and charities supporting people with HIV. I referred myself to different charities and services. I missed the support groups from London, but I was lucky that I found George House Trust, Body Positive Northwest and Black Health Agency, where I met lifelong friends.

In Manchester, I found there weren't as many people as possible living openly and confidently with HIV like those I had met in London who inspired me to be a Positive Speaker. I remember people – often people who were living with HIV themselves – didn't want to associate with me because I was open about my HIV status. This is the sad reality of HIV stigma.

Reflections on my HIV journey: seeing the bigger picture

When I was diagnosed, there were a number of courses people recommended to me. These courses helped and supplemented the support I received from charities, and I learned how to manage and cope with my condition. I also learnt about emotional, physical and mental wellbeing. They acted like a foundation of how to move on. Over the years I was supported to become a Positive Speaker, where I used my lived experience to support others and create HIV awareness. I also became a patient representative and then a Trustee at Body Positive Northwest, George House Trust, and Catholics for AIDS Prevention respectively.

Being diagnosed with HIV has really given me skills and opportunities that I would never have thought of doing in my life. Before I was diagnosed, I just lived my life. I didn't think too much about other people's problems. Now, though, I think about other people's problems more. I know as a person living with HIV you can be judged and discriminated against. I think when it happens to you, that's when you start thinking about people who are disabled, who have mental health problems, seek asylum, are refugees and have nowhere to stay. You start to see a bigger picture, that actually there are so many problems in the world, and we need to help if we can.

I'm open about my HIV status. However, when you're living with HIV, you live it with other people; your husband is part of your HIV status, your children are part of your HIV status. I don't want my family to feel burdened by my HIV status. I wouldn't want my son to find himself explaining to his girlfriend that he's negative or positive because I'm HIV positive. Many times, I have been asked if my husband is living with HIV. It has nothing to do with my husband, this is me telling you, about me.

I wasn't lucky like other mothers who came here with their children. I went back to see my son when he was 18 years old. I had planned how I was going to tell him that I was living with HIV, but it happened in a different way altogether.

He was living with my sister at the time. One day, he kept going in and out of the house and I wondered what he was doing. I was worried he was mixed up in some trouble. As I spoke to him about my concerns in relation to his behaviour, I said "You better look after yourself – do you know what I'm living with?" Although it wasn't what I had planned, that's when we started the conversation about my HIV status. He later told me he was organising a party as he and his friends had finished their A-Levels and that's why he was going out lots. I felt so much better that we had talked about it, and he was supportive.

I think it is very important to have the right conversations with our children. Our parents' generation didn't want to talk about sex. The only thing parents think about is to say don't come back pregnant. There was no information about how you even get pregnant! They don't talk to you about your feelings or your hormones, which I think is a really important thing to do as it helps you to be aware of your sexual health as well.

We are still living. I am fortunate that I live in a country where we have free access to HIV treatment and care. HIV treatment is getting better. Every year, medication is improving. People are living longer, though of course we have other health problems as we live longer. To battle against something that you know is going to be here for life is wasted energy. It's better to use that to your advantage.

The everlasting bond of meaningful relationships

Meeting other women living with HIV has created an everlasting bond. Even when we meet in different situations, we have something in common, we have this underlying connection. We look out for each other – "Are you ok?" That kind of stuff. I call them my family; I can share everything with them including articles and resources about living well with HIV. I wouldn't have met these women had things been different, as they are all from different backgrounds and countries. As a result of these connections, I have learnt so much. They have become important people in my life.

People are not just medication. I know hospitals are giving us treatment, but it is always important to connect people to charities where they can be supported. The doctors deal with the medication, but people are not medication alone.

There are lots of messages about HIV prevention and it is important to link people into support and advice services when they test positive. I met a lady who spent thousands of pounds buying treatment online as she didn't know it was free, so it is important to make sure people receive the right information and support.

Meeting people where they are

When I started working with mothers whose children are living with HIV, I realised the challenges they experience. Some think they infected their children, and they have to deal with feelings of blame and shame. So many women struggle to even talk to their children about it. I realised I did not think about all the things these mothers have to deal with. There are so many layers to living with HIV.

We had an International Women's Day celebration recently and there was a lady who came in crying due to a recent HIV diagnosis. When I shared my story with her, she thanked me for being honest as she thought she was alone in this. I've been diagnosed for over 20 years and feel like I have a PhD in HIV. I've supported a number of women to become Positive Speakers, and it has been wonderful to see how they have grown by using their lived experience to support others. I'm still working in the HIV sector and every day when I see somebody saying, "I feel better" I also feel good.

To all the women who are standing up for people living with HIV, thank you for never getting tired.

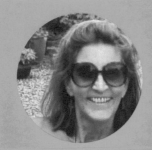

UNLEARNING LIFE: THE TOUCHSTONE OF HOW HIV CARE SHOULD BE PROVIDED

Alice Welbourn

was diagnosed in 1992, so that's 30 years ago last summer. Before that I had been living and working in Africa for the best part of the 1980s. I was doing PhD research in a very isolated rural part of Kenya and I felt really privileged being there because it was a very remote part of Kenya, but people welcomed me. They were incredibly kind to me. I was living in very unusual circumstances for people in the West, I'd say, literally living in a thatched hut with mud walls, no electricity, no running water, no sewage system, no mod cons at all, in a very traditional community. I quickly learnt that there's no such thing as a straight line in nature, apart from maybe a sunbeam, but it was just the most amazing experience. I was incredibly fortunate because it really, completely transformed my perspective on life, and all of the privilege that I have grown up with, and also gave me a massive appreciation for shared human values, because people were just so kind and so generous and so welcoming to this complete stranger in their midst.

I learnt so much from them about what's really important in life, and I've always used that experience as my touchstone, moving forward with life since then, and thinking about, well, would this policy, work there? Answer: no. Would this programme work there? Answer: no. Would this law... etc. It's just been such a valuable kind of baseline for me really. Once I finished that PhD, I was completely determined that actually what I wanted to do in life was to give something back because of everything that they'd given me.

I was able to find a job working in Somalia and went and lived there for five years. I was just so struck by the huge generosity of Somalis, and again I had massive experiences. I was working around issues to do with gender and access to resources and so on, and how gender plays such a huge role in all of what we were doing – a primary healthcare programme amongst a nomadic community in the north of Somalia, amongst other things; supporting colleagues working with street children in Mogadishu, then finally coming back to the UK and supporting people with what was called participatory learning approaches. This involved training NGO staff, really to unlearn what they had learnt in their agricultural colleges or nursing school or whatever, where they had been taught very much in a Western top-down, evidence-based science approach to 'This is what is the right way to do things,' and 'This is what you need to go and lecture community members on.' And I was saying to them, 'Well, actually, as NGO staff, it's really good for us actually, to go in and listen to community members and learn from them, because they're the experts in living there, as we haven't lived in their community,'

It was important for me to learn from them and to be using visual techniques like mapping exercises, body mapping, seasonal calendars, lots of different ways of learning from people that don't involve reading and writing. So, it doesn't involve literacy skills, and recognises that people are deeply knowledgeable about their environment and about the world around them; that education doesn't equate with intelligence; that people can be deeply intelligent and yet not be able to read or write. Similarly, people can have a high level of education and not be very intelligent. So, all of that was just incredibly valuable. In a sense, I sort of had a depth of understanding that I'd learnt from living and working in Kenya and Somalia. I was also really privileged in being able to travel on much more short-term trips, across East and Southern and West Africa, and also Asia, running these training programmes. I was fortunate enough to also to develop a sort of breadth of understanding of different contexts and different communities. On the one hand, recognising that actually, we all have more in common between this around the world, than we have differences, but on the other understanding the importance of context, and how different cultural contexts or geographic contexts or whatever have an influence in people's lives as well.

'That's nothing to do with us ...'

I was diagnosed in 1992, and the world fell apart.

In 1992, people were talking about HIV. In fact, when I'd been working for an organisation in Somalia, when HIV started first to be talked about, I actually gathered together a group of Somali colleagues who were working in the same organisation to say, hey, maybe we should start talking about this together. My boss at the time actually said, 'Well, that's nothing to do with us, that's just about people's personal lives. And this isn't something to do with work. I don't think it's appropriate that you should be kind of suggesting that this should be a work topic for discussion in the workplace.' Which was a bit of a shocker. So that was really the climate in 1992.

It was assumed that this was something that just affected the gay community or people who used drugs or whatever, and that it wasn't really anything to do with anyone else, and certainly nothing to do with women. That's not what I believed myself, but that was the sort of public perception, and in 1992 there was no medication. Among people whom it affected, there was, of course, huge stigma associated with HIV. There was that dreadful campaign on the television: the message said if you get HIV, you get AIDS, you die. Period.

Just dot the i's and cross the t's: the excitement of starting a family

I was incredibly lucky, because I was expecting a baby when I was diagnosed. I had a fantastic GP, who was a really warm lady, just a really special lady. I was fit and well and really excited about being pregnant and having the baby. And she said, 'Well, you need to come in for your tests, let's just do an HIV test as well, shall we? Just to dot the i's and cross the t's. Because I know you've been travelling in many different parts of the world.' In those days, the assumption was that HIV had something to do with other parts of the world. So, I said, 'Yeah, sure,' not imagining that there'd be anything to be concerned about.

She phoned me on a Friday afternoon and said, 'Can you come in?' and then told me that all the other tests were fine, except for the HIV. That is still embedded in my brain. What was so special was that her very first words after she told me were, 'Can I give you a hug?' So, she was instantly putting control back into my hands. Even for her to think of touching me was in itself amazing, because in those days so many people just wouldn't go near somebody with HIV without being masked up and with full PPE (personal protective equipment). Even if she'd said, 'Let me give you a hug,' that would have been incredibly kind of her, but it would have still been a sort of assumption that was OK. But she actually said, 'Can I give you a hug?' So she was asking my permission to hug me. I've reflected so often on that, it was just amazing, that instantly your world falls apart, you're completely out of control, and she was instantly putting control back into my hands. I said, yes, of course, so she gave me a massive hug and that in itself was just so amazing,

Obviously, I wanted to tell my partner and I was incredibly fortunate, and still am. I wanted to and felt confident telling him because I know so many women who would be terrified of telling their partner, the fear of violence. Then she said, 'Well, would you like me to come home with you and help to tell him?' And so she did that. That was just again, so kind of her. It wasn't like, 'Oh, well, I'm busy. I've got to see the next person in a few minutes. She was just completely clearing the decks for me and coming home with me. I was incredibly lucky, because she arranged for us to see the HIV consultant the next morning – on a Saturday morning. I mean, can you imagine? When she did come home with me, she went into a separate room and told him, while I just sat and hugged the kids.

The HIV consultant the next morning was just so incredibly kind to us both, and spent a good couple of hours with us explaining things. I continued having him as my consultant until a couple of years ago, so I feel lucky to have had that amazing support from the medical team, because I then had a medical termination (for fear that either the baby or I might die). But, yeah, just the care throughout it all, I was just so lucky, because I know so many women who have had a totally opposite experience.

Hitting rock bottom: the value of peer support

Even though they were all supportive, I just hit rock bottom in terms of self-esteem. I learnt about Positively Women from somewhere, I've no idea how or who, but I got the number and spoke to somebody. I was very terrified, on the phone and said, 'I've got HIV,' and she was an Irish woman and she said, 'Oh, yes, I've got it too.' I was just so shocked that there should be somebody else on the end of the phone saying, 'Oh, yes, I've got it, too'. That in itself was just amazing. Then I arranged to have a massage there, and that was incredible.

Before going to a peer support session there in the evening, I was walking down Regent Street, trying to waste time before going. I was literally thinking I might as well just throw myself under this bus because what good am I to everybody? Anybody? I've just brought shame on my partner and my family, even though I knew that, of course, my children needed me. I just felt so devastated. I then met Leigh, who was amazing because she was leading the group, and she described how she'd been diagnosed at Holloway, basically through the slot in the door, and how she had, there and then, decided that the day she got out of Holloway she was going to make sure that never happened to anyone else.

I just sat there thinking: who am I? How dare I imagine that I had the right to take my own life when someone like her is so amazing. So that peer support of Leigh basically completely turned me around.

I started volunteering for OXAIDS, which was in Oxford, my nearest town, and there were a couple of really lovely kind women there. Initially, I was supposed to be doing office filing, but that was utterly hopeless. I just couldn't think straight. I just completely lost the plot all the time. They didn't lose trust in me. They said, 'Would you like to become a trustee?', which was incredible, because they didn't give up on me as a hopeless case.

At the same time, through them I met another woman living with HIV in the area. Together, we decided to start a peer support group. This was in maybe early 1993. We started a peer support group in Oxford, and we were possibly the only white women in the group to start with. There were maybe as many as 12 or so, and most of the other women were African, coming from various different countries in Africa and feeling a long way from home. Also feeling really anxious that other women from their country, that somehow if they met other women from their country, at the peer group, word might get back to their own families or contacts in their own countries. It was fantastic when they came, but it was a real challenge for them.

Sometimes I would go and meet them separately outside the peer groups in their own homes or meet up for a walk somewhere, or whatever. It was just so lovely to be meeting and talking, because in those days there wasn't any treatment. To me, it was just so special to be meeting with them and connecting with them when what, for them, was a long way from home and so I just felt really glad to be able to be having that peer support, sharing everything with them.

It's such a privilege to be part of such a great group of women

I think that what has been so powerful and special for me is that I found the African women have always just been so incredibly dynamic, and vibrant, and positive, despite all of the adversity that comes with moving to England and having to cope with the appalling way in which migrants here are treated, and issues around asylum. I remember when we used to meet together in different parts of the country, those great sessions that we had with women in each of those different areas of the country, and the appalling stories that they would tell about the years of limbo, in seeking asylum here, and not having the right papers and not being allowed to work. What a travesty of justice, that they were having to wait so long in limbo without a decision being made.

People at the time were having to live in such poverty, because they weren't able to have an income of their own, and yet what an appalling waste of their talents it was that they weren't allowed to work. Yet, despite it all, they would still come, they would still be part of the group, they would still be doing so much on a volunteering level, basically, trying to make things better for their community, and for other women, in the same boat as themselves. I just always feel so incredibly grateful and so privileged to meet and to know such amazing women, over the years 15–20 years.

When finally they were able to get their papers, they just blossomed into such phenomenal powerhouses doing such amazing things. I think that has just been a real privilege to know them and to be in touch with them over the years – and thinking about 4M as well, which as a group has done such phenomenal things; thinking about back to the Manchester workshop in 2015, when so many of the women, who are really lovely women, but also very shy, very retiring, very anxious, full of lack of self-esteem, how phenomenal they all are now. Look at them now, what great peer support has done to support them to grow into who they are now. It's just absolutely phenomenal and it's just such a privilege to be part of such a great group of women.

We are all in this together: finding the right support when you need it

The whole thing around pregnancy and the right to be a mother, the right to have a positive pregnancy, is tied up with how I was diagnosed. In 4M, most of the women are African/Afro-Caribbean migrants. For me, it has been important to share those experiences because of the context of my diagnosis. We are all together in this, whoever we are, wherever we come from, but I feel particularly because I've gone on working globally and because most of the work I've done has been around sexual and reproductive health and rights, and particularly around the perinatal context and how women are appallingly treated, specifically in the perinatal period, has been the focus of my work.

I think it has also meant a lot to me on a personal level, particularly as I live in a very rural area with no local support. The 4M peer support virtual network has been a great support to me because we all, as activists, work professionally, but it doesn't stop us from needing a personal level of support. I think it's only by having that we can carry on doing what we do. I think I am lucky because I also have my incredibly supportive partner and that's a really important part of the mix. I think having really supportive friends and peers who know what it's about and can share lived experiences is also incredibly precious to me and you know it is all the kind of fuel and energy from which I can draw to do the work that I do.

You can't ignore a third of people living with HIV

We were in the right place at the right time as Salamander Trust to support 4M to grow and expand across the UK. We just happened to be able to do that and it's fantastic that we were able to find funding to have the Manchester workshop, because I think that 4M has just been an amazing creation and we're just so happy to have been able to enable that to happen. I think that has been a major achievement.

Lessons learnt: I think there is an increasing awareness and a lot of it is down to 4M, and to Sophia Forum and Positively UK as well. I mean we can't ignore a third of people living with HIV in the UK who are women. We've got to think about what does that mean in terms of appropriate treatment and appropriate support, and also the huge percentage of women from minority communities who make up that third. I think that the compass is shifting at last along those gender and ethnicity dimensions – and about time. It's fair to say that over the years we've seen increasing meaningful involvement of women living with HIV in BHIVA conferences, but I think there's still a way to go.

It would be really great to see selection criteria around meaningful involvement of women living with HIV as co-authors of abstracts. For the international AIDS conferences we've been looking at what percentage of abstracts accepted are by women living with HIV out of all the abstracts accepted, and how many of them have women living with HIV listed as co-authors or presenters. I talked about this with somebody the other day and asked if somebody could be listed as presenter on an abstract being submitted to the AIDS conference so that she could then mention that in her application for a scholarship – and she said no, that she thought that would be dishonest. I thought, oh, that's interesting! It's up to you; you decide what you want to do. I wrote her an explanation about how the current whole way of knowledge creation is a colonial legacy where basically it's academics interviewing people, getting their PhDs and sailing off into the sunset with their careers, and this happens again and again. Academics mean well and they are full of good intentions, but actually it's a completely unfair environment where so many people have done research 'on' African women or 'in African women' this and 'in women' that, as it's often described, as if basically we are all lumps of meat on a dissection table, instead of being living breathing incredibly dynamic powerful sensual beings.

I feel really strongly that women should be properly respected and ideally paid to be involved as co-collaborators from the get-go, from the whole design of the initial survey etc, through to implementation of services, programmes and evaluation. That would be great – and also, for example, we've been involved in the WHO SRHR guideline and the Canadian physicians, and women living with HIV in Canada have actually turned that into national guidelines, with a toolkit for women living with HIV and also a toolkit for physicians and other healthcare providers. We could do the same in the UK and it would be great if we could be focusing on women-centred, gender-equitable, rights-based care across the sector and to make trauma-aware training mandatory for all healthcare workers and all people involved in social care. This would make life so much better; it would be a win-win for everyone.

There are some fantastic physicians out there and we have always been good at creating the steering committee and having them on board so that we can learn together. They are having to unlearn what they were taught in medical school that 'you are the expert, you have the answers'. Obviously they are having to learn from us as well, so it's been a learning journey for clinicians, too. I just want to make it clear that I am not trying to wag my finger at them!

> Women-centred, gender-equitable, rights-based care would be a win-win for everyone.

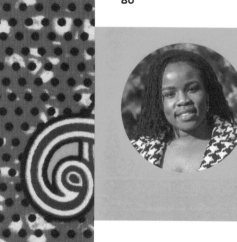

CREATIVE WAYS TO CONVEY MESSAGES: TRYING TO CHANGE THE HIV STIGMA STORY

Bakita Kasadha

When it comes to the HIV sector, I've kind of grown up within the space because I've spent my adulthood in this space. I'm a researcher, writer and poet living with HIV. I'm currently working at Oxford University on the Nourish-UK study, which looks at infant feeding decisions among women and birthing parents in the UK. I use poetry quite a lot in my advocacy work as well, trying to think of different and creative ways to convey different messages. I also do a lot of writing around identity and health, and I'm a health journalist.

I mainly got involved because I was trying to change HIV stigma. I was living with HIV and doing a lot of work through the Children's HIV Association (CHIVA) long before I was open about my HIV status. A part of me thought, if I could contribute to the HIV sector, challenge HIV stigma, it would be safer for me to live openly with HIV one day. I've always known that I wanted to live openly with HIV, but I was very scared about the reaction that I would get, so initially I wanted to get involved in HIV campaigning and the sector so that I could contribute to combating the stigma, hoping it would be a safer place for me to come out.

Whilst I was at the University of Surrey, I led a campaign called It Can Affect Anyone, with the support and help of so many students, the university and the University of Surrey Students' Union. I called HIV 'it' just to kind of illustrate the ways in which HIV is rarely named, and the stigma surrounding HIV. It was an awareness campaign and a fundraiser. I campaigned for CHIVA, and I also did some simple myth-busting things about what HIV is and about what HIV isn't.

I've always known that I was going to be open about my HIV diagnosis from the point that I first learnt about it. I think at one stage I realised I was trying to do it the wrong way round. This whole idea of trying to make the world a safer place and then try and exist openly with HIV was kind of the wrong way round. I was giving the external a little bit too much power.

As clichéd as it sounds, the change had to kind of come from within. I realised at one point that actually I would need to make peace with my own diagnosis, and that could be enough and empowering in itself. CHIVA gave me the space to do just that.

Capturing experiences and not tokenism

The HIV landscape has changed quite a bit since I've been involved. One of the key differences is 'U=U' – Undetectable=Untransmittable, a campaign led by Bruce Richman – and the fact that we now know, and the evidence is there, that if a person is taking their medication as prescribed, they can't pass on HIV sexually. That's a massive thing.

Representation has changed. When I was coming up through the scene initially, different people, whether it was trans people, black people, black trans women or young people, were having to fight more to make sure that their experiences, our experiences, of living with HIV were being captured in the mainstream, on both national and international levels. I think now, I say cautiously, organisers on national and international levels know that they will be heavily criticised if that diversity of experience isn't there. We're more visible, but it's important that our presence isn't tokenised.

I would also say, one of the key things that have changed is 'test and treat'. When I was diagnosed there was a long period of time between my diagnosis and starting medication. Nowadays, if people test HIV positive, they are advised to start medication soon afterwards. Perhaps it's a controversial statement, but I believe the delay in starting ARVs helped me with adherence. I didn't have the constant reminder of medication from daily medication. I had friends who struggled and some developed illnesses as a result of resistance or sadly died. The role of pre and post-counselling and peer support is so important.

Tokenism has been a low point for me when reflecting on my experience. There's been more of a call for diversity of experiences, and the importance of capturing a range of experiences, which can also be done in an incredibly tokenistic and an incredibly harmful way, especially for young people and black women.

Unfortunately, women continue to be underrepresented in treatment clinical trials, which oftentimes means we don't fully understand the impact of treatment on our bodies until they're licensed. A small study found an association between dolutegravir (DTG) and neural tube defects, which led to some countries prematurely stating that (cisgender) women of reproductive age couldn't take the drug. Women across the world have organised to challenge the underrepresentation of women of clinical trials. Women have always been here, and it's inspirational seeing how a few collectives of women continue to galvanise for the many.

Finding a blueprint

It's been so important to meet women and young people with HIV, through organisations such as CHIVA. There was a time when hearing HIV on the news was enough to ruin my day and I wasn't sure how I would survive this. Seeing people like 'Uncle' Marc Thompson and 'Auntie' Angelina Namiba living openly, cheekily and forcefully with HIV gave me a blueprint to know there could be another way.

I think it's very important when there are different groups and different key populations that are affected by HIV in different ways that we continue to work collectively and that we don't work in silos. I think sometimes we do end up working in silos based on different identities, so that's something that I would really like to be done differently. I think probably, going forward, one of the things that we need to do differently is I think we spend a lot of time preaching to the converted, talking to ourselves. So one of the reasons why I say that is, for example, in the National AIDS Trust in 2021 report HIV: Public Knowledge and Attitudes, the results were pretty stark and highlighted commonplace stigmatising views of HIV and lack of awareness. For me, it felt a bit like, 'Wow, I don't know if our messages are really getting through about how much HIV has changed to the people who need to hear them.' Maybe as a community we're potentially spending a little bit too much time just talking amongst ourselves when we might need to work on other public health campaigns.

You don't have to be the poster girl

I am currently in a state when I'm realising that I don't need to be all things to all people. In a talk I once said, 'Tell your story on your own terms. You don't need to cut yourself wide open to share it.' So, to my younger self, I say this: life does get better, and you made the right decision on sharing your full HIV journey with the whole world, but at the same time avoid being led by your ego. I think across all types of social movements, individuals are propelled into the limelight, and I have definitely become one of those individuals, but it's important to say yes to things because they are the right thing to do. Stay close to community, rather than being led by ego.

The work I'm doing on Nourish-UK has the potential to have a big impact (watch this space). I'm so proud to be part of the study team.

In 2016 I decided to come out and be open about my HIV status. It's been a high for me personally. It's worked just because I feel like I'm no longer living a double life. I believe that's had a direct contribution to my achievements. In 2022, I won the Young Investigator Award at the 12th International Workshop on HIV and Women, and it felt incredibly poignant being a young black woman doing that. I wasn't expecting it and felt really emotional receiving it.

In 2016 I co-edited a special collection with Dr Shema Tariq from UCL called HIV and Women, where are we now? It was a special collection between the Women's Health Journal and the Therapeutic Advances in Infectious Diseases, which are both journals from SAGE Publishing, and it was just phenomenal to be able to curate a publication exploring prevention, looking at access to treatment, quality of life before and beyond diagnosis, looking at cisgender issues, and looking at transgender issues from adolescence to menopause and beyond. It was such a privilege, and I'm really grateful to Shema for bringing me on board that and advocating to SAGE that the journal should be co-edited with a woman with lived experience, and more broadly in terms of highs, just seeing the advances in policy, and in terms of law and also just the global and collective push, on the global, international, national and community levels for better quality research for trans-inclusive research, for research disaggregated by gender, and just the importance of making sure that research impacts so much.

On health equity, I wish for a world where I wouldn't even need to be an HIV advocate, where it just wouldn't be necessary because our humanity would already be recognised – and when I say 'our', I mean all of us who are disproportionately more likely to live with HIV. Because our humanity would be recognised, there wouldn't be these disproportionate rates of health inequalities, and we would already be getting the care and the respect that we deserve.

I want a world where there is equity and where there's equality, and everybody has the right to be treated with humanity.

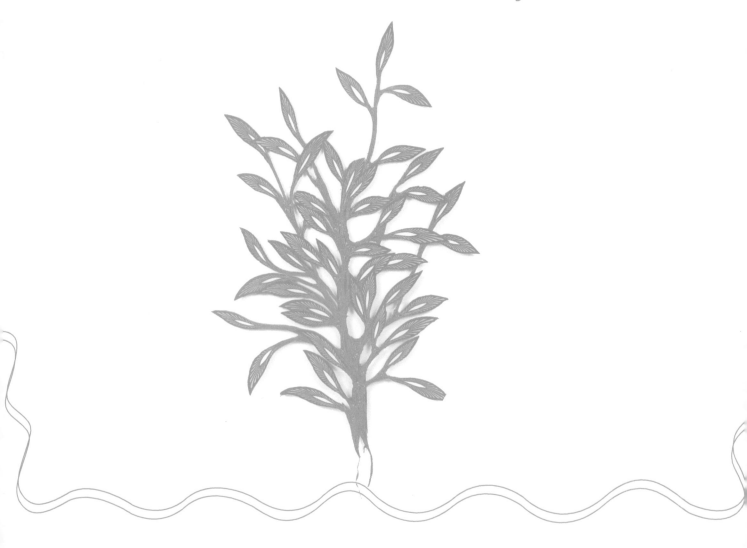

WELCOME INTO MY WORLD OF LIVING WITH HIV: THIS IS MY JOURNEY OF LIVING POSITIVELY, OPENLY AND FABULOUSLY

Bisi Alimi

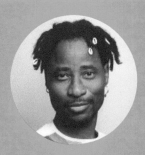

was diagnosed with HIV on 4th May 2004, and we could stop there. However, that sounds a little too boring, so let me welcome you into my world of living with HIV.

I was born and raised in a very religious home. At a very young age, I came to the realisation that I was different. That was the 1980s in Lagos, Nigeria; there were no words like 'gay'. We knew about homosexuality, and it was not such a nice word. I remember getting called 'homo', which is another word for a detergent in Nigeria, so you will hear kids singing this song when they see me coming.

Before my diagnosis I was an actor. I was also in the university studying Theatre Arts. Acting was my safe space; I guess because it gave me the opportunity to exist in an illusion. At a young age, to escape bullying and harassment, I created an alternative universe where I could be anything I wanted to be, so studying theatre art was just me taking my illusion to another level, which helped.

Acting on TV brought me fame, money, respect and access to many things I lacked as a kid, and it also brought me great pain. This pain made me search for a community of likeminded people and this was how I got into the gay scene in Nigeria.

An encounter that changed my life: the start of my HIV journey

It was in 2002 and my best friend died. The death of Ibrahim changed everything for me. His death not only made me depressed and scared for my life, but also it was a reminder of the silence that permeated the gay scene of Lagos at that time.

Every week in Lagos during the early 2000s, young, brilliant and good-looking gay men were dropping dead like dry leaves in autumn. It was a terrifying moment for every one of us.

We knew what was happening but we were too scared to name it. It was like the film Candyman, where if you say his name three times in the mirror he would appear. We felt the same about HIV, if we said the name it would appear. It was not just that; there was also the shame and stigma within the gay community in Lagos.

Before Ibrahim died, I had the chance to spend a few minutes with him in the hospital, and that encounter changed my life and started my journey into the HIV world.

It was a heterosexual world: no space for gay men

Sexual health education and support were only for heterosexuals. There was nothing, absolutely nothing for gay men. It was also the time the ABC policy was being pushed by the Bush administration: abstain, be faithful or use a condom. These messages targeted heterosexuals, so growing up gay in Nigeria gave the illusion that HIV was a straight people thing, and you couldn't have it if you weren't straight. The homophobia and stigma associated with HIV fuelled the spread of the virus among gay men.

Treatment was also not encouraging. I remember the early days of HIV treatment, such as the early drug D4T (stavudine) and other toxic drugs that deformed many people living with HIV.

One of the lowest points for me was realising I was HIV positive and asking what that meant. I had to go back on set, where I was working as an actor after my diagnosis, and this was a big thing for me. I was already struggling with the secret of my sexuality, and here I was dealing with being positive.

I remember the day I got diagnosed, and the first word the doctor said was, 'This is the beginning of another journey for you.' I couldn't see that. All I could see were my late friends who had died of the virus. At that moment, I knew I had met my Waterloo and I would never get through it. I was 29, a TV star, and just about to lose it all.

As I walked out of the testing booth, I had people waiting for me with hands wide open, and this was the best foundation for anyone just newly diagnosed. I live today because of these foundations.

Luckily for me, I had a great support network. These people were there the day I got diagnosed and were there with me for years, supporting and encouraging me on how to deal with everyday challenges, and I think this made the most significant difference in my life. Looking back at my life, I realise I am where I am today not because of things I did differently, but of the selfless people who were there for and with me.

The role my friends and healthcare provider played was beyond ordinary; they were my superheroes. Finally when I met my boyfriend, who is now my husband, I struggled with disclosure, and I had to read a lot of books and other peoples' stories to help me have the conversation with him, and when I did, what he said after that made all these pictures perfect. He looked into my eyes and said, 'Thank you for telling me. This means the world, and I want to be part of this journey with you.'

Nothing makes sense

When I got my diagnosis, I remember feeling like I was learning amid a problematic experience, which is challenging. You are learning things, clearly, and yet nothing makes sense. I remember, a friend once said I was lucky, and I couldn't put his argument into context. Lucky for what? I am alive, but glued to a drug for the rest of my life. As I've grown older and wiser, these messages from different people have started to make sense. HIV has taught me a lot about life and living.

Eighteen years after the doctor told me, I was optimistic. I learnt to trust science more. I developed tools to handle the survival guilt and develop the skills of telling my own story in a way that empowers others. I have also learnt that taking my HIV meds can just simply be eating breakfast; it is not a big deal.

I live my life in public,
so you don't have to
live yours in private.

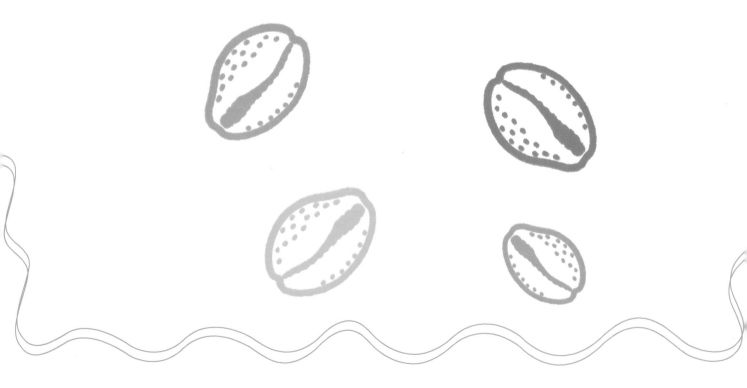

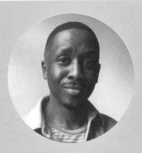

NAVIGATING HIV AND ADOLESCENCE: A HOME AWAY FROM HOME

Bryan Dramiga

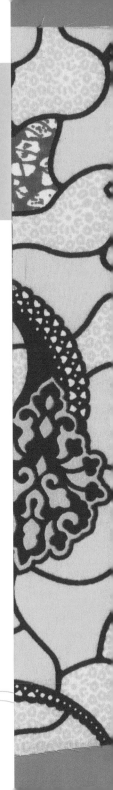

Life before

Great Ormond Street is etched into my fondest memories; yes, it's a hospital, and a reminder of my illness. However, it was strangely a place where my mother and I could spend quality time without the interference of my siblings. Every three months, on a Friday, we would drive into the city. We would laugh, sing and inbetween belting out Chaka Khan and Tina Turner hits, we would catch up on what was going on in our lives, what we wanted to do, what we wanted to achieve and she'd reinforce the hopes she had for me.

I remember the colourful wards in paediatrics, the nurses and their warm smiles. I remember how they'd encourage me, enquiring to see whether today was the day I was ready to take blood without the numbing spray. I would always start off, resolved, that this was the day and then fear would settle in and I'd plead for them to spray the whole thing. The discomfort of taking blood was dwarfed by my mother's reassurance of how brave I was. Having my choice of lolly and animal plaster sweetened the deal. The hospital visits were our day out. Those childhood memories served as a positive foundation for all my hospital trips in the coming days. That was life before I knew about my HIV status.

Life after

At age 11, the clinician informed me of my status and I was quickly referred to the peer support services offered by Barnardo's, the children's charity. Peer support was amazing. It acted as a temporary safe place for me to express anxiety, concern, confusion and other emotions regarding growing up with HIV. I met with people my age who were different, but understood the loneliness, the anger and more importantly the silence of HIV at home. Peer support slowly became a home away from home where I could express my feelings and be met with understanding or at the very least a listening ear.

Welcoming newcomers

By age 14, peer support had evolved from some of its earlier members attending with their negative siblings (the affected) for support, to now the group solely being comprised of young people living with HIV. Newcomers were slowly being introduced, apprehensive, some silently observing for weeks before having the courage to share. 'What difference does it make? Sharing all of this stuff? We're not normal. Even with meds who would choose us? If you were negative would you choose this?' These kind of comments were pervasive, although they had the potential to impact morale negatively, it was important to let the sharing party vent their frustrations.

The newcomers' ideologies were met with positive rebuttals. Yes their concerns were justified, but they needed to be reminded that we have the power to shape our realities and be the change we wish to see. Peer support was a place where we could vent, share our challenges, when one of us wanted to take the next step and share with a negative friend, family member or partner. We could and would often use the time to encourage and role-play potential outcomes. This would go on for years and the group would share victories, losses, tales of unrequited love, rejection, summer romances and first kisses. We grew up together, charting the murky waters of sexual and social maturity.

The team at Barnardo's utilised my extrovert personality and willingness to interact with new people. I met and supported many of my peers learning English and those who struggled navigating a bigger social group. This time enabled them to develop the resilience needed to combat bullying and created a safe space where they could share their concerns. The social workers equipped me with tools to run workshops and activities with my peers.

Reflections: peer support over the years

Peer support doesn't end. We'll always need someone to talk to and I believe there will always be someone available to connect with. Looking at what I would hope to be the last generation of young people living with HIV, I am relieved to see that the key lessons have been shared with various organisations that work with said young people. It's evident in the growing sense of shared optimism towards the ending of stigma, a sentiment shared not only by the young people, but also their parents.

Whilst many of the peers I've grown up with have navigated and established their HIV identities, building careers from their status, forming families and loving relationships, some still have all of that and yet battle with internalised stigma that surfaces in issues related to adherence. It saddens me to hear of my peers still hospitalised as they wrestle with issues outside of their HIV, be it familial, financial or spiritual.

Many of my peers who had found a home in the HIV organisations that provide peer support had no such home established where they spent most of their time. Peers poured their livelihood into activism but failed to shape an identity outside of it. I've come across peers who reached a point where they wished to sever ties with any form of peer support and had reached a point to say yes, I am OK with who I am but I am not an activist. This is to be expected and accepted, as I don't believe the goal was ever to make all of us activists, but to reach a point where we could all navigate society with a sense of belonging, purpose and strength.

Yes, there have been many successes that have resulted in a number of us beating the odds, remaining undetectable, edging closer to this unspoken goal of normalcy. I've had to ask myself, though, what is normal? Being undetectable? Being an activist rallying against stigma at every opportunity? What of those who would and will still struggle with adherence until the end? Are they not normal? I've come to the realisation that peer support will never end because we're all different, and we're all at different stages of healing, learning and understanding. It could take 10 years, 20, 40, until a cure is released, even longer. It doesn't matter how long it takes. There will be people there to support and those in need of supporting.

The main ingredient to successful peer support? Empathy. I can't stress this enough. My experiences have helped me nurture my compassion for people with stigmatised conditions. If I didn't have HIV, I doubt I would be as understanding or liberal. It's given me a deeper insight into what it means to care genuinely about people. HIV has opened my eyes regarding how I can best relate to people as I navigate life. That's the most rewarding thing, building bridges, so that I can help my positive peers take their eyes off themselves and on to someone else who's younger than them or those going through something they can help with, not to invalidate their emotion, but to put themselves on pause to help someone else's healing. If we can just try to commit to the healing of others, by lending an ear or giving encouragement or sharing laughter, that's the healing we might need ourselves.

HIV at home: silence in the African community

I can only speak from my experience and echo that of my peers in so many words. There's no secret that the majority of young people who attend the CHIVA summer camp have come from African households. HIV is not an African problem, it's a human problem. However, the way it's been dealt with is very African. If you're offended by what you're reading, you're more than welcome to discuss solutions to the issues I'm about to divulge, if you wish to just complain, get in line.

Within the African community, speaking about HIV openly is difficult, and creating a safe space to talk is nigh impossible. In my pursuit of belonging, culture and manhood, I looked to my elders to get an understanding of what it means to be a real man. I looked to address the issues I had in myself and pit them against a model of real manhood and see where I came up short. I had a number of questions regarding traditions and values. I wanted to grow and gain experience from those that came before me. The only issue was no one was available to have a real conversation. Every man I wanted to speak to was dismissive and simply wished to break bread and make trivial small talk. I am in no way painting every single African male elder with the same brush. However, from my lived experience and upon speaking to my peers, this is somewhat the norm.

I've got a number of relatives whom I have found to be positive, not through them but through whispers. There are people in my family who are rumoured to be positive and people know that I'm positive, but nobody comes to me and says, 'Oh, we know you're positive. We've always known.' We know these things are happening, but we don't want to talk about them.

It is an issue within the African community because it's not discussed in our households, even with our affected peers adjacent to us. I could be alone in my house. There's no sense of true family. We want to cover up and never discuss the undesirables, in order to keep the wants, needs, desires, insecurities and anxieties of those at the seat of normalcy fairly intact and unquestioned. This is how I've processed this information, not maliciously but pragmatically. I mean, I get it. If I were them, where would I even begin to navigate the conversation?

Blue-sky thinking? It would be great to come to a point of understanding, to break bread with people who hold opposing ideologies, to come to a point of understanding after arguments have been shared. That would be a massive thing within African communities, although I don't believe there's genuine empathy. I believe there's this idea of culture, but no one can actually explain it to me, so it comes across as this fluid ideology of an antiquated tradition colliding with western sensibilities.

To conclude, there's a beauty in Africa that escapes me. I love Africa, the landscape, the people and the food; but the value systems and the ideologies and the traditions that keep us stuck? I don't know. I know that certain traditions are rooted in age-old principles that uplift the human experience. However, some traditions make me feel ashamed. I would love to cherry-pick, as culture shouldn't be static; it should grow and change. Well, I'm only talking about the African community's attitudes concerning the HIV sector anyway. It could save a lot of people from dying in isolation.

Our lived experiences are different, and how we perceive and process the world is different.

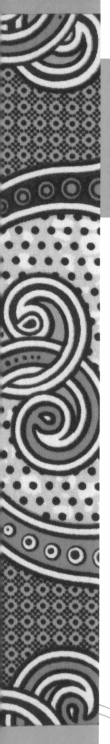

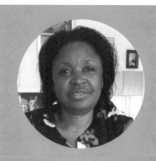

VOLUNTEERING TO SUPPORT MYSELF: THE HIDDEN DISEASE OF OTHERS

Eunice Sinyemu

I started my teaching career in 1988 at Njase Secondary School in Southern Province of Zambia where I taught History and Zambian Languages. Like most people, prior to my HIV diagnosis I was a free-spirited individual, very ambitious and always looking out for opportunities to improve my life and further my education. I moved to Scotland in 1994 to join my then husband and this was a great opportunity for me to further my studies, something that I had always wanted to do. This is the year that I was diagnosed with HIV.

Despite my diagnosis, I continued pursuing my ambition of furthering my studies. My interest changed from education to business administration and eventually years later I obtained BA Honours Degree in Business Studies.

Confused and in denial

After my diagnosis my life changed, as would be expected. I was confused and in denial. It was the denial that later made me to start wanting to understand what HIV was and how I could help support other people. At this point I did not want any support from anybody, because I believed I was not HIV positive. I started to look for organisations that worked in HIV. I went to an organisation called SOLAS in Edinburgh. When I got there, I boldly said I was not HIV positive but wanted to help those who are. This was the beginning of my real nightmare – the reality of being HIV positive sank in. I started understanding what being HIV positive meant and in a way I was volunteering to support myself and found solace in this.

In 1994, HIV in Scotland was very much associated with gay men and those who injected drugs. There were very few African diagnoses then and HIV was not openly talked about, and as a young African woman I felt alone because I could not talk about my HIV with anyone. The majority of those who were HIV positive were white gay men. There were very limited treatment options, and you took what you were given, basically. There wasn't much information on HIV. Although support was there, it was very hospital and respite-based support. During this time I saw so many AIDS-related deaths. The HIV movements that we see nowadays were almost non-existence. It was a hidden disease and a lot of times many people believed it was a disease for others not them. Many of us were gripped with fear of dying and not talking to anyone about it was the worst. The treatment that was there was aggressive with numerous side effects and people took it because they had no choice.

Opening up and living with HIV

When I started being open about my HIV status to my children and selected friends this really started to help. I have experienced a number of different relationships that have helped over the years. One of the lows of living with HIV has been my changes to my body due to treatment. This happens a lot when I go shopping for clothes; I come out of the shops feeling really low.

Being linked into great services, including HIV support services away from the hospital, has helped a great deal with my ability to stay well. Having a number of friends who I can call anytime has been of great help. The support from my son has also been invaluable.

Self-care, supported by adhering to treatment and keeping doctors' appointments, is also an important lesson that I have come to learn in the process of being HIV positive. Another lesson I have come to learn is that you can be who you have always wanted to be before HIV diagnosis, while still making vital contributions to the HIV sector. We don't all have to be involved in the HIV sector. HIV should not control one's life, but rather the other way round

In life, I have learnt not to judge other people but accept everyone as they come. We are each unique in our own way.

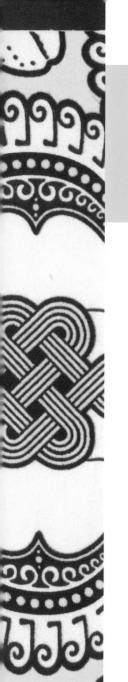

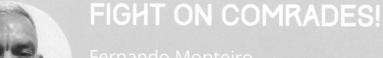

FIGHT ON COMRADES!

Fernando Monteiro

was on my first year of university, studying International Relations when I was diagnosed with HIV. Until then, I was a young person trying to be the best version of myself while navigating being gay in a very homophobic culture.

This was 1991. Lisbon was an adopted city because I was displaced by war from Luanda, Angola, from where my family fled in the mid-1970s. We lived in Brazil before settling in Lisbon in the early 1980s. Although the gay community came out of the closet in the late 1980s, Portugal was still an unwelcoming place for queers. From my early teens to my being diagnosed, it was a long period of trying to fit in, being rejected for being gay and a migrant.

At the age of 16, looking much older, probably because I had to grow up quickly while trying to integrate, I discovered the gay scene and made my first gay friend, who is still present in my life today. Clubbing became not just a celebration of our queerness but also an escape from traumatic experiences of rejection socially and at home. We looked for validation and love in all the wrong places. Sex became a way of relating to others and seeking acceptance.

In 1988, the Portuguese broadcaster had an evening dedicated to the emerging AIDS crisis. For the first time I was exposed to what was going on in New York and Africa. I watched a series of programmes with my family and my gay friend, in my parent's living room. Although we were in silence as we paid attention, I keep being distracted by my thumping heart beating against my throat as fear slowly crept in and took hold of me. When my friend and I went to bed, we talked about the sadness of it all and were scared that we might have caught AIDS. Straight away, I told my friend: 'What's the point of doing an HIV test? We will die nevertheless.' We kept talking through the night, comforting each other.

Time stood still

In the spring of 1991, I had a dramatic presentation of shingles and ended up in A&E. The dermatologist sat down with me and asked me if I was gay and had unprotected sex. I said yes to both and he explained that I was too young to have shingles. Therefore, there must be something wrong with my immune system and I needed to test for HIV.

I remember having an out of body experience when I came back two weeks later to receive the test's result. The minute the dermatologist told me I tested positive, I flew up from my chair and crashed against the ceiling's consultation room, where I had a bird's eye view of me sitting in front of the doctor. I crash-landed back on my seat when he told me that I probably had six months to a year to live. Time literately stood still and I spent most of day crying.

The HIV sector in Lisbon was very small. There was the Liga Portuguesa Conta a SIDA (Portuguese League Against AIDS) and Abraço (Embrace). Those were mentioned to me by the psychologist who supported me after my diagnosis. I immediately volunteered with both, as I wanted to meet others going through the same experience.

At my first infectious disease appointment, I met a petite woman, an angel-like figure, whose kindness was so mighty. Silvia was her first name and she told me, 'No one can tell you exactly how long you have left. Therefore, focus on living one day at the time and make the most of it.' She suggested I take AZT, the first drug available to treat HIV. I accepted.

Although, I was linked in with good after-testing care, services weren't geared up to support people living with HIV. We didn't have specialised treatment centres and we faced terrible discrimination within healthcare. We were prevented from accessing dentistry, and finding a surgeon to operate on us was like searching for a needle in a haystack.

I spent seven months being referred here and there, but was always put on waiting lists – which was a polite way of saying, 'We won't treat you' – until my psychologist heard from a sexual health doctor that there was a female surgeon who didn't mind operating on people living with HIV. This visibly queer surgeon met me with her nursing assistant for a pre-assessment appointment. They were so compassionate and respectful. They spent part of the consultation apologising and agreeing that more needed to be done to support people living with HIV, who were waiting endlessly for surgery.

We were also banned from health insurance and mortgages, and had our careers terminated if our status got out. We had the media portraying us as monsters and murderers. Therefore, we needed a lot of support to mitigate the impact of this on our already fragile mental health, as HIV affected disproportionately those who were already discriminated against, namely gay men, migrants and intravenous drug users.

Standing tall: the healing power of peer support

Although there wasn't a name for it in those days, I knew the healing powers of peer support, because of the unconditional love and support I received from my gay friend(s) when I grappled with homophobia and self-acceptance. Around the same time of my diagnosis, I got involved with LGBT rights and met Nick, a South African man, who proudly stood up in one of our meetings and shared he was living with HIV.

His dignity taught me that I should always hold my head high and never let others put me down because of my HIV status. He became a good friend and role model. Funny enough, we found out we were neighbours, which made us even closer. We spent long nights chatting after dinner. He read gay publications and current treatment updates in English. He had access to things I didn't. He told me about ACT UP in America, stressing that the way forward was through gay militancy and HIV activism. Sadly, within a year Nick was dead, my first of many losses to AIDS.

Despite so much adversity, we, people living with HIV, and our allies came together to fight back. We were crucial in setting up services that people enjoy today. As a young gay man, I would have loved not to have experienced that level of trauma, but at the same time I am so proud for having been part of that inspiring movement of people who stood up for our rights, and showed that compassion and love for one another will always carry us through the toughest of times, and that collectively we can achieve greater things.

In early spring of 1996, I relocated to London with one suitcase and dreams of becoming the next hot filmmaker. When the plane circled London, I was surprised by the big sprawl. A friend told me I could register my care with the Kobler Clinic, Chelsea and Westminster Hospital. I was pleasantly surprised by the number of resources available. There were leaflets about everything, volunteers giving you tea and cake, well-appointed premises and the staff were so nice, respectful and compassionate.

Visibly proud gay people worked in there, which made it so comfortable for me. Every health professional I came in contact with spoke to me in such a casual, friendly and direct way, a far cry from what I was used to. Unfortunately, I couldn't get my meds prescribed because I was already on combination therapy, which had just been approved in the UK but wasn't available yet. Luckily, I brought six months' worth of meds that lasted until the clinic could dispense my combination.

Adjusting to living in the UK

As I integrated in life in the UK, I started using support services available at my local drop-in centre, River House Trust. Once I had my first AIDS diagnosis, I had so much support from my clinic, social services and the HIV sector, which was literally a lifeline.

The HIV sector was a much different affair from today. The need was different and definitely more complex, as people living with HIV were tiptoeing between life and death. Combination therapy did change the health and life expectancy of people living with HIV, but at the same time it pushed us back into the biomedical model of care. We need to constantly challenge this idea that meds are a panacea, because we know that treating HIV is a very complex affair.

It still bothers me that most of the services are localised in London and that we have disparities of care and support across the country. Living with HIV in rural areas is a very different affair from in the big sprawl, and within London we have a postcode lottery, that restricts access to services by funders. Unwittingly, we are creating exclusion zones of care and support, where our brothers and sisters can't be properly supported and consequently end up struggling unnecessarily.

In early 2012, I lost Alan, another great friend, advocate and HIV activist, one of the founders of Blackliners, who was so instrumental in my acceptance of my black heritage. His loss left me devastated and plunged me into depression. At a counselling session, the therapist suggested I volunteer and reconnect with the HIV sector. I heard of UK-CAB and decided to attend one of its meetings, where I met the then chair, Silvia Petretti.

Although I was friends with positive women, I had never met such a glamorous, empowered and articulate woman living with HIV. Her activism sparkled. During the lunch break, I approached Silvia, who was so welcoming. She suggested I attended their

Taking Part programme, a series of workshops to empower positive people. I am so glad she asked me, because volunteering with Positively UK was such a momentous thing for me and opened so many volunteering and professional opportunities.

At Positively UK, I met more beautiful and wise women, who helped me further reconnect with my African roots and showed me the long road that women living with HIV still have to track in order to be respected, accounted for and properly included in treatment research and care. My sisters made me understand that their struggles are mine too and that I must use my 'gay man's privilege' to advance their cause, fighting alongside them, like they have done alongside gay men for eons.

Reflecting on a life lived with HIV

Looking back to my 31 years of living with HIV, I am mesmerised by the wondrous developments in HIV medicine, but we mustn't let up. People living with HIV still suffer from discrimination and self-stigma, are still disproportionately affected economically and in some cases have poorer health outcomes than the general population.

Women living with HIV are being treated with drugs that weren't developed for them, as their inclusion in medical research is still debated today. They are disproportionately affected by poverty and gender-based violence. So are our brothers and sister who are transgender and have to negotiate the intersectionality of stigma.

Therefore, we mustn't be complacent, because HIV treatment is not just about accessing good and free healthcare here and abroad. Only a holistic approach that puts the needs of the individual at its heart will suffice. We must carry on fighting until we eradicate stigma, so that our brothers and sisters can live freely and be the best versions of themselves. We can only rest when we rid the world of stigma and provide everyone with the best treatment options, independent of where they live.

If my 21-year-old self could have looked past his immediate bleak future, he would have been able to see that his life would have its meaning and purpose enhanced by HIV. Looking back, that's what this 53-year-old gay man has realised. If I could, I would send my younger self the following missive: 'Fight on, comrade. HIV will take and give in equal measures. It will be a hell of ride, but you will be stronger.'

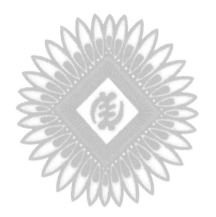

Let's bathe in the glorious light of those who paved the way for us and let's fight on, comrades!

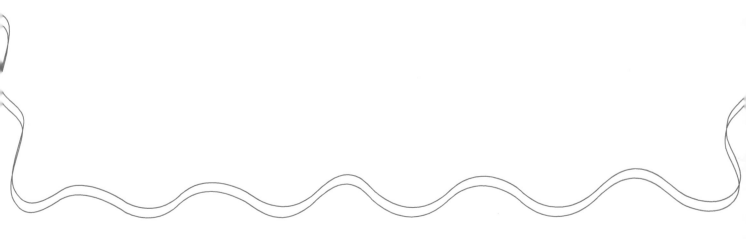

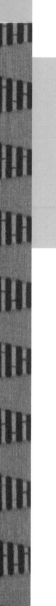

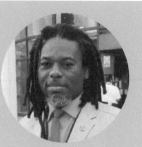

EVIDENCE OF A SINFUL LIFE: ACCESSING INFORMATION TO HIGHLIGHT THE TRUTH ABOUT HIV

Godwyns Onwuchekwa

Except for a mention of HIV in one biology class in secondary school, my first real encounter with HIV was through the church. I use the term 'real' because it was the first time it registered. This is because the context was steeped in stigma and oppression. These issues constantly stir me into action.

It was 2002. I was 23, lived in Maiduguri, north-eastern Nigeria, and was active in the Anglican Church. The women's group in the church – Mothers' Union and Women's Guild – hinted they were bringing a motion to deny church weddings to anyone – mainly men – living with AIDS. (The acronym HIV was rarely used.) They believed that AIDS was evidence of a sinful life.

Being quite involved in the church's activities, from choir to youth fellowship and church council, I was privy to some critical discussions. My archdeacon had taken me on as a protégé and co-opted me into the church council, where I was the youngest member. The council met once a month on a Saturday morning. This meeting was also where I first subtly revealed my sexuality.

As the secretary, I said very little during meetings because I was busy writing and taking the minutes, which the council preferred in verbatim style. When the matter of this AIDS motion came up, I was confused because my incidental knowledge from my biology class a few years ago made it clear that HIV was just another infection like others. One thing I remembered from my school lesson was that HIV could also be transmitted in other ways than sex, the so-called sinful activity, as if no one in that room engaged in this sin. Focusing on taking notes, I made no contribution to this agenda item. Most importantly, I knew nothing beyond the one paragraph of notes from secondary school, so I needed to read up and prepare.

Luckily, I worked as an IT officer for a bank, in charge of the branch. My position gave me access to the internet, a privilege in those days. I started researching and learning about HIV. At the next meeting a month later, when this point came up for discussion, we needed to conclude and give support as a church so that our synod delegates could be sure which way to vote, but there were no doubts which way that was going to be. Nevertheless, the archdeacon had a democratic leadership style and would allow every matter to be discussed thoroughly, to ensure that everyone had felt heard, and for this he was also reluctantly liberal in so many ways.

It was my chance to air my view, although as the secretary I should have concerned myself with taking notes and only taking part in votes. However, on this day, I indicated my interest to speak. It was the first time I'd formally spoken in the meeting. I stood up, took out my small work diary, opened it and addressed the meeting. I gave them statistics and anecdotes I had picked up online from my research. I told them about treatment and management of the condition and that the disease is not only carried by men, as was the approach for this impending ban. My contribution was more of a lecture than an input. Everyone listened candidly and appeared shocked. I didn't expect what followed; I was put on the podium, so to say, and questions fired at me to explain this and that. Before long, I realised I wasn't even half prepared for this, but I lived to fight another day (the next meeting), and it became my first victory. I convinced my church not to vote for this ban. Sadly, they only decided to abstain from the vote. It was pragmatic. I doubt anyone voted against the motion, but at least someone consciously did not vote for it.

My curiosity for HIV knowledge

It dawned on me that even doctors in Nigeria in those days, like across the world, knew little about HIV. However, it wasn't until I moved to the UK two years later, in 2004, that I realised this was the case.

Arriving in the UK, I heard more about HIV via my then GP in Stamford Hill, London. I continued my curiosity by asking even more questions. Luckily, as a gay man, my GP had a deep knowledge and found my interest in the matter fascinating. Within our 10-minute consultation, he gave me leaflets he had sought out for me and explained things. Living with undiagnosed fibromyalgia meant I saw him frequently for yet another change of medication because the last one hadn't worked. This repeat visit thus allowed me to learn. It was during this period that he suggested a few charities I could volunteer at, relying on the fact that I was then volunteering at two different charities, Scope and the now defunct Foundation for Public Service Interpreting.

At the same time, I got diagnosed with the very thing I was a silent expert in. I was shocked. Shocked because my reflections could not afford me the occasion on which I might have lapsed and ended up in this position. The question occurred to me: might it be that I have lived with HIV all my life? Putting two and two together, all the sickliness since childhood, the easy catching of any infection that went, the weakness, the endless pain, etc, and then my late mother's long sickness battling with heartache and eventually heart failure, swollen feet, etc, it dawned on me that I might have had a lucky escape. Considering that I was born in 1979, just in the shadow of the formal discovery of HIV, I concluded that this was my fate. My resolve only hardened with my already built-up frustration at how society misunderstood and stigmatised certain ill health.

The weight of the bulletproof vest and its fashionable appeal

What you might find interesting is that I didn't share my new personal discovery about myself with my GP. Not deliberately, but the private clinic where I was diagnosed had sent me to Homerton University Hospital, where I met a fantastic team of medics. They too discovered that there was a low fire in me needing to be fanned into flames. It was my support worker, Mona Nathan, one of the most gently inspiring, supportive and caring persons I ever encountered, who suggested I volunteer with the UK Coalition of People Living with HIV and AIDS (UKC). The team at Homerton, just like my GP, saw in me something I didn't know was there. While I was silently in turmoil, I was also strong enough to hold and face up to it. For me, the final call had arrived.

I didn't appear to need support, other than the nudge to take the step and formalise what I had long been doing and feeling, so off to UKC I went. There again, I met another set of wonderful people, many of whom became informal mentors and rooted for me. They all saw in me what I didn't imagine. It also meant that I was learning from the best. UKC taught me a lot and introduced me to good role models like Paul Clift, Mercy Banda,

Winnie Sseruma, and many others who took me by the hand step by step upward. Through these, I met many more.

A beehive of activism

At this time, HIV treatment was combination therapy, yet the emotional support was what many cited as the pillar of their survival. I gained my support from supporting and learning, and having moved to the UK to study and with no immediate family, the HIV sector provided me with a chosen family. In a way, being diagnosed just seven months after arriving in the UK led to me establishing this incredible network that remains my pillar to this day.

The landscape was so active. A lot was going on. Services were everywhere; support was personal and open to all. The grassroots were attuned to the difficulties faced by people living with HIV. There were newsletters for every audience. Events happened repeatedly, and training was delivered on prevention in many places. The beehive of activities meant that there was no lack of what could be done, from simple one-to-one support to programme development and policy initiatives. Everyone tucked in, and for me, the busybody, I was back in my element. I did not just volunteer with UKC, but at my clinic in Homerton, I also flipped from being supported to becoming the one member of staff sent to other patients for informal support. I was still studying, working at a restaurant, volunteering for three organisations and singing in a church choir. I couldn't get enough. I just wanted to change the world at the snap of a finger, but that's what you do as a 20-something-year-old.

The landscape I joined with my HIV activism, was firing up anyone and provided a fertile ground for anyone who dared to fight. At least, that's what I felt; there was a buzz. Within months of joining, I was being tipped for jobs, sent to run training and invited to join various working groups. These eventually are the building blocks on which I stand today.

Finding a safety net: mentors, managers and meaningful relationships

I didn't start ART until ten years after my clinical diagnosis, having become an orphan just before my 17th birthday and now living in a foreign country alone with no immediate family and no access to any state support as an international student. The team at Homerton were my safety net, including helping me access financial support for food, since most of my earnings went into my studies. Additionally, just like I refused to come out as a gay man, I applied the same principle to living with HIV, being unashamed of it and yet taking the position that I owe no one any explanation. I reveal it in instances where it empowers others, and that has a better impact.

Winnie Sseruma was a mentor I didn't deserve. From the very first day I met her at Christian Aid while delivering HIV training to the staff on behalf of UKC, she took to me like her own. She invited me to the African HIV Policy Network (AHPN), where I became a volunteer and almost immediately was tasked with organising the then annual conference on HIV for Africans and ethnic minorities. My then line manager, Walter Gillgower, invested a lot of trust in me, providing guidance and constantly reassuring me that he trusted my skill and decision.

I will not forget what he told me once during that time: 'Godwyns, the only decision you can leave for me is to sign the cheque. And this is because you can't sign it for formality and systemic reasons. But just go for it.' You couldn't ask for a better manager. So I powered on, delivering a highly rated conference that drew delegates from across the world and had a UN rapporteur as a keynote speaker. It was humbling as much as it was bizarre, but I enjoy working and organising stuff anyway. This opportunity also saw me responsible for 15 fellow volunteers, many of whom became friends.

In 2009, just four years within the HIV sector, I was going further and becoming active in LGBT activism, and the support poured in. In 2010, I set up Justice for Gay Africans (JfGA) to get the Commonwealth Secretariat to denounce publicly the criminalisation of LGBT people in Commonwealth member countries. It was at this time I met Peter Tatchell. He was a stalwart of LGBT activism who also took me under his wing and constantly reminded me that I could do it. He got me in front of the then Commonwealth Secretary-General. And also in front of the Secretary of State for International Development and into many radio and TV studios to speak. Peter's mantra was, 'You're born to do this,' or something along those lines.

When you're gone, what will happen? The role of activism

There is a new range of young activists coming up, but HIV activism remains a victim of its own success, at least in the UK. This is my personal opinion, but I always take the long view. When I asked ageing activists 15 years ago what would happen if they were not bringing new and younger people in, giving them room to shine and watching those young ones from the audience so they could correct them now, no one took it seriously.

Now we are at the point where when someone with HIV has a problem, they struggle to find a safe space to go in. Peer support groups are now like shrubs in the desert. Emotional support makes a lot of difference for every illness, and we are losing that.

What could be done differently is to rethink the approach to cultivating new voices. While our veterans were driven by need and the desire to survive not just what was a terrible pandemic but also society's ostracisation, the new diagnoses of today are dealing with undercurrent stigma that still needs to be challenged. For such, a new approach must be devised to inspire the next generation of activism. I am not denying those currently doing the work, but the more the voices, the higher the positive impact.

Working in a different space

My proudest moment was when in 2009 Positively Women handed me the role of running a fortnightly women's group. In the same vein, Homerton University Hospital gave me the opportunity to attend an antenatal class to talk to expectant parents about HIV. Some of the attendees were opposite-sex couples, which allowed the men to speak to a fellow man about stuff that was nagging them.

Subsequently, through the recommendation of Professor Jane Anderson, MAC AIDS Fund, encouraged me to run a men's group, which led me to partner Tackle Africa to deliver the project. That project went on to win funding from the Mayor of London. Being able to fit into these unique spaces gave me the stage to touch lives. Additionally, working with Body & Soul and featuring some of the young people who attended their service in the AHPN quarterly magazine was immensely inspiring for me.

Onwards from that, I had the privilege to run the service user group for the Tri-Borough (comprising Hammersmith and Fulham, Kensington and Chelsea, and Westminster), allowing me to contribute to shaping the commissioning of services for people living with HIV in the three boroughs.

Beyond that, I worked with organisations across the UK, travelling to deliver training and workshop. In 2011, I won the Vodafone World of Difference Award to provide training for people living with HIV who had been out of employment for a long time. I am proud that most of the participants in the training programme I created with AHPN went on to return to work. It has been humbling to contribute in such small and subtle measures.

We need grassroots voices. We can't leave it all to organisations and policymakers. Real lives need real solutions, not statistics and theories.

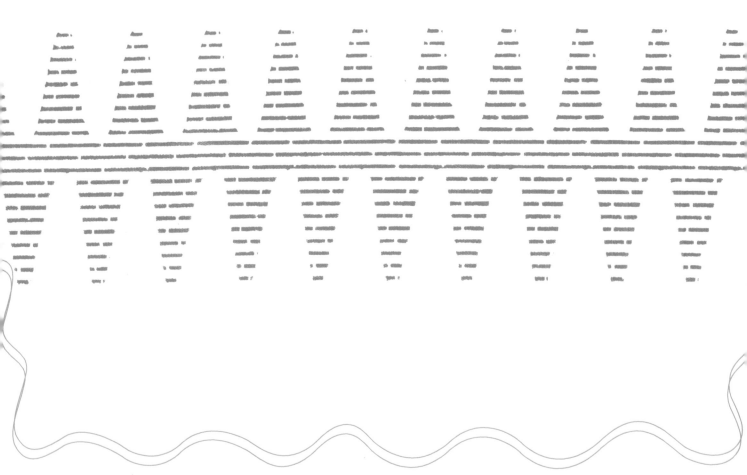

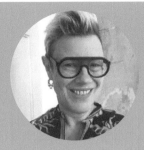

BALANCING ROCKS

Jane Shepherd

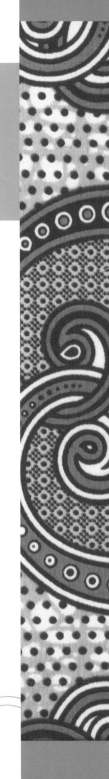

I left London for Zimbabwe in 1987 with a partner who wanted to make a film about the musician Thomas Mapfumo. I was fed up with Thatcher's Britain and a bit in love with the idea of liberated Zimbabwe with its cooperatives and collectives. It felt a world away from miners' strikes and signing on the dole. When I was later diagnosed with HIV at the Kobler Clinic in 1990, I went back and forth from Harare to London in a whirlwind of activity, trying to raise awareness about HIV and challenge stigma. I did radio interviews, designed t-shirts to raise money for Mashambadzhou – an AIDS palliative care centre in Harare – designed posters for the Zimbabwe AIDS Counselling Trust and exhibited at the London Lighthouse. I met amazing people doing amazing things, like Kate Thomson and Jo Manchester at Positively Women, and Angelina Ndlovu and Lynde Francis in Harare.

In 1992, I took the offer of teaching graphic design at Harare Polytechnic and decided not to go down the path of HIV advocacy. I couldn't do both; to live openly with HIV and teach would have been impossible, and the job suited me. I could avoid explaining anything to my family – there were no internet or mobile phones then. If I fell ill and died no-one would know why. The clinic told me I had eight years to live and my contract was for two years. I would just plan for the next two years and figure out the rest when those years were up. And then my partner committed suicide. I returned to pack up our Brixton flat. He was 28 and all his worldly belongings fitted into a black bin bag. I went back to Zimbabwe and made it my adopted home.

Struggle

Over the decade, illness crept up incrementally but always seemed manageable. Each ailment was something explicable. Shingles, gingivitis, herpes, teeth abscesses, dysentery, stubborn coughs. Each time, I put it down to bad luck (I should never have eaten that gazelle stew from a roadside café in Mozambique), stress (if only I could get a phone/car/ boyfriend) or lifestyle (those polony rolls from the kiosk, all those beers and late nights still drunk at dawn). I didn't want to know about AIDS and avoided reading about it. There was no effective treatment for HIV so there didn't seem much point. Would it have helped to know that I could go blind or demented, contract TB in my bones or get thrush all the way down my throat and into my lungs like poor Precious, my friend's aunt? She couldn't swallow in the end. Vera and the other aunties went every day to Harare Central Hospital to spoon feed her; they sat with her while she slowly starved to death. I told myself over and over, people do not die from this, whatever 'this' was at the time. I will get over it. I will survive if I can just live 'positively'. I was endlessly looking for alternative therapies and a place of inner peace where finally I would do yoga, eat healthily, stop drinking. Next week, I promised myself. Next week I'll quit smoking, staying out too late and living on peanut butter sandwiches. But like a bug spinning on its back, I just couldn't get upright. It was exhausting; the slightest movement, a wobble, a shift, would knock me off-kilter.

Surrender

Just before 2000, I had a long bout of diarrhoea that almost killed me. My boyfriend's grandmother travelled across town to visit me. It was a long way to come so I knew it was serious. I was lying on the bed reading when she arrived. 'Ambuya has come to say prayers for you,' the boyfriend said, as surprised as I was. 'She says everyone back home is very worried.' I wondered why they were so worried. Did they suspect I had AIDS? Or being white, was I exempt from the 'short illness' that so many succumbed to? I had got thin so quickly. My body had burnt up any fat first and then moved on to my muscles. I looked like I had AIDS.

She asked me to kneel beside her on the rug. We sank stiffly to the floor, hands pressed together, exactly as I had done as a child in my bedroom in Portsmouth. It now felt strange and awkward to be talking to God in my adult bedroom. As soon as the prayers were done, she promptly picked up her bag and left. We walked her up the drive and showed her the hamerkop nest in the fork of a coffee tree. 'And look, we also have a beautiful owl,' I said, turning to face the house. It was huge, an eagle-owl. It had been perched on the roof for weeks. 'Maiwe!' She clasped her hand to her mouth and looked long and hard at us. 'That thing can only bring bad luck', she snapped. 'Get rid of it.' I knew what she was thinking but I couldn't afford to believe in the power of omen or curse. Prayers, I would take.

I thought I would recover and go back to my normal life. I sort of did, enough to go to work but I was so tired I had to sleep under my desk in the afternoon. My boyfriend left me, I think he knew the end was in sight. I applied to do an MA in the UK, ever the optimist. I knew I could start treatment if I returned but I was so confused after all the years of expecting to die and then not that I felt invincible. Looking back, I was deluded, resistant, afraid. I remember being scared of treatment because I'd heard that the drugs were dangerous if you were not monitored by HIV specialists. At the time, I didn't realise this was one of the excuses used to prevent the roll-out of treatment in Africa. Despite there being so many people living with HIV in Zimbabwe and everyone touched by illness or death, no-one talked about it and there was little information. The only time I attended a support group, someone confessed they were going to commit suicide and a woman cried at the loss of her child. I found it too traumatic to return. Without meaningful peer or clinical support, my mind had created an alternative reality that both propelled me forward but in the end nearly finished me off.

Before I left for the UK, I joined friends on an ecology workshop. Each night we stared up at the immense spangly wonder of the Milky Way. In the day, we spread out, choosing a tree to sit under to meditate. Mine was a munondo, I pressed my nose against the tree and lay my cheek on its rough bark. I thought I heard it say, 'It will all be OK.'

On the last day, we took beers and climbed a small rise to sit on the granite rocks, glittery with mica, still warm from the day's sun. I pressed my palms against the rock, soaking up the heat. When I raised my hands, I could feel vibrations, that the air was not empty, that there was no difference between my skin and the air. I held my hands up in surrender, they hummed against the landscape, the blue hills, ochre soil, the huge sky. My muscles, hair, bones, virus, blood, leaves, trees, blades of grass all just molecules and atoms, dancing to their own tune, pulsating, resonating.

We are not a single story
with a single ending.

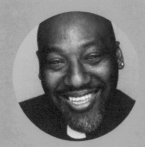

QUEER FOLKS: FINDING THE RIGHT COMMUNITY FOR ME

Jide Macaulay

When I was diagnosed with HIV in January 2003, I was 38 years old. Before then I'd had many privileges and some challenges. In the decade before my diagnosis, I had been in a painful heterosexual marriage, and I was experiencing lots of anxieties and a mental health crisis. I worked for the Crown Prosecution Service and for PricewaterhouseCoopers following the completion of my law degree and professional training. I was highly involved with the local African Independent Christian Church where I had been recognised as a senior leader within the fold. The Nigerian community was my home. I came out as gay in 1994 and it was difficult to find the right support for black gay men and also to find the right inclusive Christian community. I was excommunicated from the church and the Nigerian community became toxic and homophobic.

After finding the LGBT community, which was largely white and male, I started to get involved with organisations such as GMFA and other small groups such as BIGUP. I served GMFA as a trustee and volunteered as a sexual health worker. These experiences brought me closer to more knowledge and information. I also wanted to find the right community for me. I later discovered a pocket of black queer folks interested in faith and socialisation, mostly south of London.

I started working in the HIV care sector in a voluntary role, but later became more impactful after my own diagnosis with the virus.

The fear of being punished

When I was diagnosed, many people I knew with HIV had either died or were very ill. I had feared HIV, even though I was helping to share knowledge about its awareness. The HIV landscape was filled with a high level of stigma, shame, denial and lots of discrimination. When I was diagnosed, I was angry. I was truly ashamed that with all the knowledge I had stupidly allowed myself to become infected, and that led to a number of years in denial and self-discrimination and self-stigma. At some point I had internalised the idea that God was punishing me for my homosexuality.

Treatment was good when I was diagnosed, although the peer support structure was very poor and this was problematic for me. It took six years post my diagnosis to find the appropriate peer support that I needed, and in reality this support was not as good as what I had hoped for. All the time the peer support lacked the cultural and traditional needs of a Black African homosexual man.

Reconciling my faith

Post diagnosis my zeal to live right led me to reconcile with my faith and sexuality. I began to gain trust in God regardless of the hateful religious views. In 2009, six years after my diagnosis, I had the opportunity to listen to black folks living with HIV who are also part of Christian leadership in Cape Town South Africa. I began to come to terms with the fact that I am not alone, when I found a peer support group at Positive East in the same year that ran workshops over a 12-week period for newly diagnosed.

One of the hardest things was the stigma I faced from friends, the rejection from sexual partners when I disclosed my status and the religious abuse around HIV. I would fear going to the clinic in case I saw other black folks. For many years following my diagnosis I hid the truth and facts from my friends, colleagues and family members.

The power of social media

The ability to disclose my HIV status publicly has been a great help and I did this on social media on World Aids Day 2018. Advocating for others and providing peer support services, including HIV mentoring, has been a great part of my journey. Coming across organisations such as INERELA+ helped to put things in perspective for me. As a result of my public disclosure, I have been able to advocate for the right HIV peer support for other black gay men and developing a holistic approach for gay men living with HIV remains a highlight of my journey towards wellness.

Lessons are rarely learned in this situation. What I will say is that people's experiences change them. I have become more compassionate as a person. I have great love and respect for myself and others. I recognise differences that may set people apart. These low times don't last unless you allow them to hold you in captivity. What has held me together is my faith in God and my inner strength to take me from a low place to higher place of celebration. It's important to know that effective treatment means you become undetectable and unable to pass on the HIV to sexual partners, which is worth celebrating and a boost to my mental health.

Faith and HIV

When reflecting on my life, it is important to take the negatives and make them positive. My contribution to the HIV sector is both personal and professional. Being visible about living well with HIV as a Black African British, openly gay Christian theologian and an Anglican priest is a major achievement. I have been involved with major sexual health campaigns for years and remaining consistent in providing information and supporting many others through their own journeys.

Low times don't last unless you allow them to hold you in captivity.

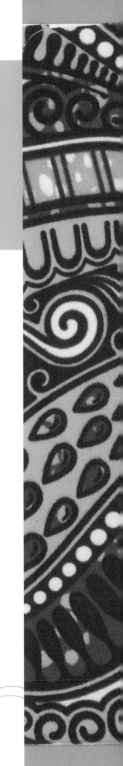

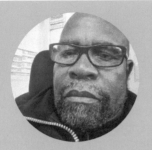

FAILURE TO THRIVE: THE DEVASTATING EFFECTS OF HIV IN THE ZIMBABWE COMMUNITY

Lazarus Mungure

I am originally from Zimbabwe. I came to the UK in 2000. When I was still in Zimbabwe quite a few of my workmates and very close relations contracted HIV and had very prolonged illness. A lot of them succumbed to AIDS due to infections. A lot were emaciated because their bodies failed to hold the food they were eating. I know lots of acquaintances who first went blind before they died. In the 1990s there was no effective medication to control the progression of the disease. Some were fortunate to be offered the trial drugs that were available, some stopped taking the medication when their health improved and for others the progression of the disease was very rapid.

What we were seeing then was the signs of infection appearing in new-born babies. They often didn't grow well and experienced a multitude of chronic ailments that didn't respond well to treatment. They would generally die a few months after birth. People callously referred to them as failure to thrive (FTT). The trend was generally that the mother would subsequently fall ill. They would survive the debilitating illness for a while, failing to respond positively to medical intervention. For some families the deaths followed different permutations, resulting in many young families being annihilated. That left a massive burden on the elderly, who often had to fend for the orphans.

This became the most fearsome disease of the era. Contracting HIV meant certain death. Church-sponsored clinics bore the brunt of caring for the terminally ill. As far as I was aware there was no effective cure for AIDS, as it was generally referred to.

Moving to the UK: a change in my pattern

When I came into the UK, I was resident at Hatfield in Hertfordshire. I used to commute to London for work every day. I had a full-time job, initially from 8am to 5pm. There came an opportunity to join the shift team, which meant a more challenging routine. I then started at 7am to 7pm on day shift and 7pm to 7am night shift. This affected my eating pattern. I noticed I was beginning to lose weight. I had to punch new holes in my belt to hold my pants up. Physically I was feeling quite well, didn't miss a day at work due to illness. During that period two people I knew were admitted into hospital with an HIV diagnosis. They were very ill and I visited them. One was at St Thomas in Waterloo, and the other was at King's Hospital. After a long time they both recovered.

In the summer of 2002, someone I had a very intimate relationship with became seriously ill and was admitted into St George's Hospital. The diagnosis was that they were suffering from opportunistic infection because they were HIV positive. I decided to have myself tested for HIV. Even though I didn't feel unwell, I was slowly losing weight. I was very apprehensive for a couple of weeks while I awaited the results. Since I wasn't feeling ill I hoped the results would be negative.

Eventually I got the results; obviously they were not what I'd hoped for. I was shocked to learn the state my body was in. The viral load was extremely high and my CD4 count was 29. The consultant was very surprised. He had never seen a case like me. I was informed that I had to start taking medication immediately. In my condition, I was told if I fell ill my chance of surviving was very low. Given that I was in full-time employment my consultant and I had to work out a combination of drugs that wouldn't cause disruption to my work routine. I underwent many tests to check for TB and other infections. I was given a combination that would have the least impact on my routine. Unfortunately, one of the drugs had to be refrigerated. That posed a challenge as I was sharing a flat with a stranger, but I was fortunate to have a small fridge in my bedroom, so I wasn't forced to disclose. I immediately set out to find my own accommodation, where I wouldn't have to share. It was fortunate that I lived within walking distance of the hospital. Because of the very low CD4 count, I needed more frequent monitoring.

Vibrant hope, amongst a battery of treatment side effects

The hospital staff referred me to a support group, ACIA (African Communities Involvement Association), in Mitcham. I got a very big surprise when I attended the group. The leader of the men's forum was someone I knew from Zimbabwe. When I had seen him last in Zimbabwe he was in a critical condition. I was pleasantly surprised to see the transformation. He looked well and vibrant. It gave me a lot of hope for a full recovery.

I wasn't to enjoy the benefits of this support group for long. I was transferred to work outside London so I wasn't able to access the services of this group. I still received treatment from the same consultant and hospital to maintain continuity in monitoring.

Within a few months my viral load came down considerably, but the CD4 count struggled to go up. In agreement with my consultant, I volunteered for clinical trials of new drugs. In one trial they were monitoring the distributed fat imbalance that was triggered by some HIV drugs. The other trial was monitoring the effects of certain drugs on bone density. The last trial I was involved in was seeing the effect of mono therapy for people who have been on medication for a long time and had a high CD4 count and undetectable viral load. To date I have now been on mono therapy for over 10 years. The advantage is the reduction of the pill burden and the side effects caused by combination therapy.

The biggest challenge I had with my first combination was that one of the drugs gave me the runs. I couldn't take a pee at a urinal without running the risk of soiling my pants. I remember one incident when I accompanied someone to Gatwick airport. I went to the toilet for a pee. In the process at the urinal, I felt the urge to break wind, but lo and behold, I felt a slimy stickiness flowing down my bum. I quickly went into a cubicle to check; my briefs were soiled. I quickly took them off, wiped off as much muck as I could. I went out to the washbasin and washed off the shit then went on the hand dryer and dried my briefs. When they were reasonably dry, I put them on, then went back to join the people I had accompanied. I was worried that I would have to explain my long absence, as I did not want to disclose my HIV status. So, I just fobbed them off. I'm not sure what they made of my excuse. It was a very unpleasant situation. From that time, I avoided using the urinal each time I wanted to pee.

Feeling compromised to share my status and the liberation that followed

After a couple of years my work contract ended, and I applied for an extension to my visa. This process took a very long time. I wasn't allowed to work, so was on a very low income and was forced to share accommodation. I was still on the medication that required refrigeration. I was compromised and had to disclose my status. After a while I found that very liberating because I didn't have to look over my shoulder about my HIV status to those I associated with. Because the Home Office was dragging its feet deciding the outcome of my visa application, I was classified as an undocumented immigrant. I began having stumbling blocks in accessing medication. Every time I visited the HIV clinic, I was sent to the foreign department to register before I could see the consultant. This resulted in me receiving very large bills of several thousands of pounds for treatment and medication. It was a very trying moment, being denied the right to find work and having no recourse to public funds. I was really at a loss what to do.

One major challenge was the negative attitude of many in the medical fraternity. When I went to register with a new GP, they wanted to know what other medications I was taking. I indicated that I was on HAART, the reaction I got was surprising, to say the least. The receptionist concluded that I had a heart problem, I jumped the waiting queue and was ushered to the doctor. It was only there I was able to clarify that I was on highly active anti-retroviral treatment that the doctor calmed down. A very irritating practice when I visited the hospital for intrusive examination or surgery was being put at the end of the queue even though my appointment was booked for earlier than other patients, because I was HIV positive. As a positive speaker and advocate I always challenged this. Once when I was admitted into hospital for knee surgery when I'd torn the patella tendon the nursing staff noticed my HIV drugs and wanted to take over the administration. I firmly refused to give them, as their routine didn't tally with my self-medicating timetable. I have heard others have been bullied, resulting in medication being given to them at times that didn't conform to their adherence routine.

Advocating for change

I began volunteering for SLAWO (South London Advocacy and Welfare Organisation), an organisation that advocated and provided temporary shelter for victims of domestic violence. I helped organising meetings for the forum for men who had suffered from domestic abuse. I later joined the AHPN. I was a very active member of its projects, Vital Voices and later Ffena, the network of Africans in the UK living with and affected by HIV. I participated in advocating for universal access to HIV medication. We made several representations to several committees at the Houses of Parliament. I was glad when eventually the bill was passed. It is still in force to date. In the end I didn't have to pay those hospital bills.

Another project that I was involved in was the development of the Christian and Muslim faith toolkits. I volunteered to pose as a Muslim Imam on posters distributed to many hospitals in the UK. I received several phone calls from people who knew me, wanting to know if I had converted to Islam. I was an active contributor to the Stigma Index project, which collected evidence of cases of stigma experienced by HIV positive people in the UK. This also resulted in a presentation at the Houses of Parliament with celebrity Annie Lennox.

As part of my advocacy work, I have had the opportunity to work with members of large pharmaceutical companies such as GlaxoSmithKline, Abbot and Gilead, articulating the challenges people on medication experience. I am confident that the contribution of the focus groups helped in the development of drugs with better efficacy and fewer side effects. This promotes better adherence and more positive outcomes. I have attended BHIVA, CHIVA and the International Aids Conference.

One major challenge in the early days of the HIV pandemic was the prosecution of many for onward transmission of the virus. It put the onus of disclosure to a new partner on the diagnosed person. It became a focal point of the campaign to decriminalise HIV. We have been fortunate now that we have made great progress and have the U=U campaign which aim to communicate how effective treatment reduces the number of new infections.

Even though there are several new revolutionary drugs that are given at much longer intervals than the daily cocktail of drugs, the vaccine and cure are still the elusive holy grail.

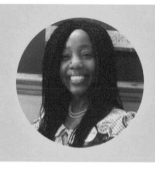

THE SKY IS THE LIMIT: GRIEVING FOR THE LOSS OF MY OLD LIFE

Laura Dayit

I came to the UK to study for my Masters in Business Management. I had always wanted to work in community development and at the time I was thinking about becoming a social worker. As I was completing my second Masters degree I was working as a project worker at an ex-offender service, helping ex-offenders back into the community. I secured a job as a social worker, but because of visa issues the job got withdrawn. I moved back to Peterborough. I was just in the process of starting to work with an agency and was trying to figure out what I was going to do next, then the gift of HIV came knocking.

I received my diagnosis in hospital and at the time the only people I saw were professionals. I just kept asking them, are there other people actually living with HIV? Can I see them? They were very supportive in my journey, they visited me and wanted me to eat. I feel that because I started my journey with other people living with HIV they are more like family. They also made sure I got the professional support that I needed. The social worker that visited me said, 'I'll give you the address of the place where you can get support,' which was Positively UK. I remember the first time I went there, and I was walking around and could see that people were living with HIV. I thought, this is the sort of place that I'm looking for.

I wanted to be part of the community, so I volunteered to do the peer mentoring programme where I met lots of different people who helped shape my journey. These people helped me to learn more about what it meant to be living with HIV and were instrumental in my decision to move from Peterborough to London.

When I got diagnosed, I did not realise what it was or that it would change my life so much. I remember that I went to the airport to pick my father up. I said, 'I think I'm having a heart attack.' I must have looked really bad as he called the paramedics. The lady on the phone asked if there had been anything that had happened to me lately, so I whispered that I had previously had pneumonia – then I paused and said that I had recently been diagnosed with HIV. She advised me to go back to the clinic.

On Monday, I went to the clinic, where I was seen and offered counselling. During the counselling session the counsellor said to me, 'Do you realise that your life has changed and that you now need time to grieve your old life?' I've had to learn to stop sometimes and grieve, and then move on. I have learnt over the years to stop and allow myself to process what is happening and listen to what my body is telling me.

I feel like HIV has given me perspective in life. As a result of my diagnosis, I have met wonderful people and created lifelong friendships with people that I have met along the way.

Advocating for others

Sometimes we need someone to advocate for us, which involves providing spaces to have these conversations. It is about supporting people when they feel like running away or going through a difficult time and encouraging them to live their life on their terms. Stigma is the biggest challenge when it comes to people being able to do this.

My frustration is with the ones who don't get seen, who have so much to give, and the value that Africans bring to the HIV community is huge. We are a big part of the community, culturally; our background is a community. We've always been a community. We build communities. That's what we do. Look around, anywhere you go and they're talking about community, then that's where it's largely made up of us. We have so much that we need to contribute to the narrative, but sadly enough, sometimes there is no data to support our experiences. We build community because we understand the value of community, but sometimes we can be quite naive in the sense that we get used without realising that we're being used.

Working at a grassroots level, we are the frontline workers who are often dealing with lots of issues. We talk a lot about intersectionality and what this means when trying to provide support to people. Immigration is still a big thing. We are migrants and sometimes the process of being here and getting used to being here can be quite lengthy and complicated. I was reflecting recently about how immigration affects our representation, how it affects our ability to be seen and how it intersects with stigma.

What a lot of people end up doing in the HIV community is volunteering. People don't realise that if you're volunteering when you go to apply for immigration it's actually a plus for you. I think it is important to recognise the value that is provided when you attend these spaces; and being part of a community and part of a support group, that is your value in showing up. When you share your story, when you share your time, that is your value.

The people who shape our stories

I have had so many relationships that have helped me on my journey that I sometimes I sit back and think, wow!

I remember Chris Sandford, who has now sadly died. I went to Bloomsbury clinic to do my 'recently diagnosed' course, which was over three weekends. I would go every Saturday and we would spend the day there. In the early days that relationship helped me. He was the person that mentioned to me about the 4M Mentor Mothers network.

Years later, it was like a dream when I was invited to do work for 4M. At this time 4M was still part of the Salamander Trust, where I was a volunteer at the time. I was really eager and enthusiastic. I just wanted to do a good job. The invitation to be part of this project was a real highlight for me.

My journey with 4M has just been incredible. The progress that I made with Angelina Namiba and Alice Welbourn has been phenomenal – the fact that as soon as I was allowed to work, I started getting paid and then I got more responsibility. Even though it was work, the support that I received really helped and shaped me. That's why for me it feels like family.

I remember the activism training where I met Paul Decle. Being part of Positively UK and doing the peer mentoring training and getting involved with Project 100 [peer mentor training programme], which led to attending conferences and forums, has really shaped my HIV journey. All this enabled me to start the support group in Peterborough supported by Paul.

Throughout my time in the HIV sector, I have been involved in a number of different things. I took part in the Catwalk4Power. I've worked with Positively UK in different roles, and I've also worked with UK-CAB (Community Advisory Board). Central to the work I have done is making people realise that you can have a life with HIV and being part of a community is important. I think for me, that's the most important thing. I know that things have changed slightly now in the sense that people are not necessarily meeting in rooms. People are busy living normally, but when we connect and feel a sense that you have got involved that is really powerful. I think the biggest thing that Africans have contributed to the UK HIV response is community, as that's who we are, one big community.

Nobody can tell your story how you can tell your story.

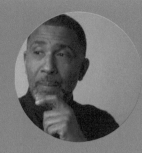

HITTING THE GROUND RUNNING: PROCESSING MY HIV DIAGNOSIS THROUGH EMPATHISING WITH OTHERS

Marc Thompson

was born and raised in Brixton in South London. My Caribbean parents were young when they had me and I lived a free kind of existence as a young kid growing up in a pretty stable, secure upbringing. My mum was certainly OK about me being gay when I came out. I think after I came out when I was 16 and left school, I just hit the ground running.

I tested positive for HIV in November 1986. I was a patient like most of us were, and had no inclination to get involved in any of the work at the time, because, I was dealing with myself. Around 1992, after going to the Landmark as a service user, I started to go to a black gay men's group called Let's Rap, a bi-weekly discussion group where the aim wasn't just HIV and sexual health. It was around community development, community building and connecting black men with each other.

Within that, there was a lot of work around safer sex and HIV prevention. What drew me in was that there had been nothing provided for me as a young, black, gay man, so I didn't want anybody to have to go through the things that I was going through. It didn't make sense to me that other people didn't understand how to prevent HIV. I wanted to share the information, although I didn't come out about my HIV to the people I was working with in these groups. In some ways, deep down inside, I've reflected on this and see it was an opportunity for me to process my own HIV, but it was also an opportunity for me to what we now call reducing stigma. It was an opportunity for me to try to address stigma by educating people, because I thought, well, if I can educate these guys, then the next guy that I meet in my personal life may not be so stigmatising. It was that kind of ripple effect that I wanted to create.

A stigmatising time

The first thing I have to say is that I was plugged into HIV care really quickly. It was in an STI clinic, but they were well equipped to deal with what was then unknown and unusual, but I felt safe and held there. I felt my clinical needs were definitely being met. In the wider world, it was frightening. It was a really stigmatising time. There was quite a lot of vocal violence towards people who had HIV or AIDS, so they didn't want to be open about their status in the wider world outside of clinics or HIV services.

In my community of black gay men, there was a lot of fear, a lot of stigma. There was a lot of gossip about people who might be positive, but really we were just scrambling around in the dark. When you look at the wider media landscape, it was awful. Everywhere you looked, newspaper reports or headlines certainly weren't sympathetic. They had no empathy for victims or for people who were affected in any way. It was quite a distressing period in those first five or six years until I found my feet.

Initially, I didn't see anything that spoke to me or black folk, at all. Whilst I was actually conscious of the need for it, I didn't engage in stuff, because I didn't see myself there. I think the other thing was that I didn't know many other people who were really my age when they were diagnosed; I didn't know many people my age at all. When I went to places, everybody was older than me, or it felt like they were, but when you're 18 or 19, anyone over 22 seems centuries old.

One of the first places I got involved in was Blackliners, around 1989. I went along to, I think, the very first volunteer meeting at a place in Brixton. Then we set up Let's Rap and then Big Up and then we had to respond outside of the mainstream, because the mainstream wasn't explicitly addressing the needs of black communities.

Anger, gossip, friendships and love: the highs and low of living with HIV

I was angry at my community for a long time, because I felt I was a subject of gossip. I was not held and not cared for by a lot of people. I was really frightened. Every time I dated somebody, it would be knots in my stomach, because I didn't want to tell people, to disclose to people, although I practised safer sex. So I didn't have sex with people. That was really, really tough. That was probably the lowest time for me, constantly going through these periods of wanting to tell people I fell in love with.

I remember my first significant boyfriend. I'd had boyfriends before, but with my first really significant, serious boyfriend, I hadn't told him about my HIV for about a year. He kept wanting me to go for a test. Eventually I was like, I've already had a test and it was positive. It was just awful. We stayed together, but the hurt was palpable. That was probably one of the lowest times for me. Losing friends was always hard, because you just felt that was around the corner for you.

One of my highs was creating Big Up in 1995. Black gay men responded to it and I was surprised by that. Our logo was a silhouette of a black man with dreadlocks with his top off and his fist in the air in a circle. Big Up was set up by two guys, Patrick Scott and Clarence Allen. Clarence had worked with me at Let's Rap; Patrick was a positive man from Birmingham and he volunteered for Blackliners and for GMFA.

Blackliners was set up as a direct response to mainstream organisations not meeting the needs of black communities. GMFA was set up around 1990 in direct response to mainstream organisations not being explicit about HIV impacting on gay men. This was a time where the health education authorities started to put out lots of messages around how HIV affects everybody. GMFA was saying that HIV affects gay men and we have to talk about that. Patrick felt that black gay men were falling between the cracks of both of organisations, because neither of them were meeting the needs of black gay men. To cut a long story short, he got a small amount of funding to provide culturally appropriate and specific advice, information and support for black gay men around HIV, for those affected and those infected.

My role was as the first Project Coordinator, which started in September 1995. I remember just sitting on my first day crying at the printer, because I'd never really used a computer before and didn't know how to work a printer. Within a couple of months, this thing exploded. We had 25 volunteers and three members of staff. We were putting out campaigns in bars and clubs. All of our stuff spoke to black men.

I joined the Terrence Higgins Trust (THT) in 2004, and was recruited to be its Programme Development Manager. I was leading all the national campaigns, and for me that was a huge leap because of the organisation and because it was a golden age of health promotion. The first thing I did was put out a monthly magazine. Every edition before had white men all the way through it. The first thing I did was say there was going to be a black boy on the cover. All the ads I did after that included black men, or we didn't do them at all.

Ensuring that the African voice is included

The work around Africa communities always felt like the poor cousin. I remember when I started at THT, we had one officer at Gray's Inn Road; at one end was the African team and the other end was the gay men's team. The gay men's team was probably twice the size of the African team. Admittedly, we had more money, and that was due to the nature of the issues being experienced within the African community at that time. The gay men's work felt much more professional. It felt like the top shelf, and the African team had some work to do.

Finding relationships that matter

When considering the relationships that were important to me throughout my HIV journey, I can probably identify three. I think the first one would be my relationship with Landmark in Brixton. The centre was important because it provided me with a safe space for a few years when I needed it the most and introduced me to a community of other positive people. It definitely reduced my isolation.

The second one would be my long and everlasting relationship with Will Nutland. He was first my manager. He was also a partner when I was at Big Up, then he became my manager at THT, and much later he became my business partner.

I think the third one is my relationship with the women that I met at Positively UK when I started working there in 2012. The reason I say that is because prior to that I had worked for women with HIV at a distance through the work with NAHIP. I didn't really know many African women and I'd worked with positive women. When I went to Positively UK, it changed me. Because of my mum, I have huge love and respect for black women. When I was at Positively UK, I saw the strength, the resilience, but also the love and the sense of community and sisterhood. It was the first time I'd seen women who had overcome adversity and were making great things in the world. This is probably one of my most important relationships.

My school of life and the lessons I have learnt on this journey

On a personal level, I've learnt patience and kindness. I've learnt that we can try anything, and we should. That's part of the fun, that where we can get to be really creative and try stuff. I've learnt we are all deeply flawed, and those flaws are what make us brilliant in many ways.

On a professional level. I've learnt how to think critically. I've learnt how to think like an academic, although I'm not one. I've also learnt that my lived experience is not just as a positive man, but also as a man who's black and queer and lives in this country, and has worked in this field, is worth eight university degrees. It took me a long time to get to that point where I can go, 'Actually, yeah, this working class boy from Brixton with one or two O-levels is pretty damn smart.

We deserve better: dipping my head into the African world

One of the first things that motivated me is that I am a Jamaican but I am a man of African descent. Way too often it's almost like there are gays there and there are Africans there and it's as if an invisible rule exists between us. I am an African man. We deserve better. I wasn't seeing that because I occupy this space of the gay mainstream world and then the black gay world.

When I dipped my head into the African world, I could see what could be achieved. When I saw some of the people who were managing the African work, I thought, oh no, no, no, you've got to go, because you are not very good at what you do and we need better. I remember very clearly, going down to Reading and it was a training run by African Health Policy Network (AHPN) and facilitated by Sigma around increasing awareness when working with queer communities and I went because I felt that the African communities needed to know that, and it would improve practices. My motivation in life has always been that black people get the best that we can.

African men and women have fought tirelessly to get a seat at the table. In the late 1990s and early Noughties, it was very Bob Geldof, very paternalistic for Black Africans: 'Here you go, we will help you, we will do this for you.' I think what our generation did was to say that, actually no, we are mature, we are educated, we are smart. We are not just here to get your handouts, we want to drive policy, to drive campaigns. We want to be in charge and most importantly, to be in charge of resources, meaning money, because there was that mistrust that Black African communities and organisations were going to piss money up the wall. We all went, no, forget that, you need to take us very seriously. Our contribution, our generation of Black African and Caribbean in the sector moved it forward, so those people who were in power had to take notice of us.

I think the resource, The Knowledge, the Will and the Power was an incredible document. When that document came out we had a strategy, we had a framework. What we didn't have was money to put it in place, so I think that was definitely a great, powerful contribution. I just think it's a shame that now we don't have the National African HIV Prevention Programme (NAHIP), we don't have fresh, young blood coming in. That's the same in the gay sector, so it's not just unique in the Black African community. Black African community work was already two steps behind, and now, without that new young blood coming in, it's four steps behind.

The Life and Knowledge toolkit for Muslim communities was also a great tool. On the back of that – and I am sure someone else will say this – the pregnancy work that happened was important, and I know that Salamander Trust was really instrumental in this. The fact that there were so many Black African women being diagnosed or having positive children at the time became an impetus for change, and a push for women living with HIV to say, 'I can speak to women in my community in a culturally appropriate specific way.' That completely changed the game.

In terms of work with African communities, one of the things we lack in this country is a specific programme of work targeting Black African communities. The national programme, for example, is a one size fits all. The London programme is one size fits all, too, and doesn't acknowledge the specific needs that we have as Black communities who are impacted by HIV. That needs to be recognised, as currently it means we don't get results, there is no research into us and there's no policy about us, so I think that it's a real shame that there is no programme for Black African communities in this country. It's just a mess.

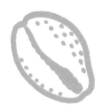 We are all deeply flawed, and those flaws make us brilliant.

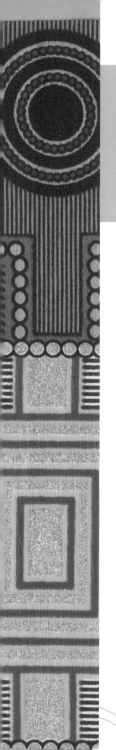

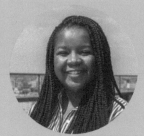

THERE IS NO LIFE BEFORE HIV: GROWING UP LIVING WITH HIV

Mercy Shibemba

have always lived with HIV. For me and many others, there is no life before HIV. Looking back, there are dozens of memories from my formative years that make me wonder why I hadn't realised sooner. However, my lack of curiosity in that regard makes me smile. In many ways, that was a gift to myself. I got to live a (somewhat) beautifully ordinary life before I knew about my HIV status, and for that I'll always be thankful.

Growing up, I was usually sure about things, probably a bit too sure. I could proudly map my way from A to B and be confident that I could get to whatever goals I wanted to reach. (I often wonder what 10-year-old me would have thought if she knew what was to come.) The three letters H, I and V hadn't really been considered in any of my plans ... Of course, this is something everyone feels. Nobody plans for this.

Survival was probably the main reason I became involved in the crazy world that makes up the HIV sector. I think for many people there comes a time when you recognise that this journey is a tough one to do alone. The joy of being known and understood is something I have in abundance because of the community of people living with HIV.

As I fumbled my way through my teenage years, I often felt trapped by the idea that this virus was something that would halt all of my plans. I always knew that my life would not be cut short by HIV.

The joy of being understood

I won't forget how affirming it was the first time I ever met another young person living with HIV. I remember catching the train from Cardiff and how the cold winter air made me regret my choice not to pack a warmer coat. Off I went to London, unsure of what the weekend would turn out like. It was such a surreal experience. These people I had never met all seemed to share the experiences I only ever knew to be true myself. It was like looking in the mirror.

When I met young people living with HIV they just got it. I didn't have any explaining to do, just knowing looks, laughs and deeply felt sighs of exasperation. I wasn't the only one. They all knew the ins and outs of what it's like to grow up with HIV in a UK context. It started me on a journey that I could never have dreamed of. My only regret was that I hadn't been brave enough to do this sooner. Well, alongside not bringing a warmer coat. I'm forever grateful to the CHIVA family who made that possible for me and so many others.

I have been grateful always to have had access to medicine and a range of clinical staff who are a credit to their disciplines, a reality I hope to be true for all people living with HIV one day. However, I was sure that my hopes had died a sorry death. That I was going to live the rest of my days under the shadow of what could've been. I am enormously grateful to have been proven wrong, time and time again.

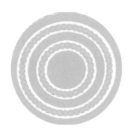

There comes a time when you recognise that this journey is a tough one to do alone.

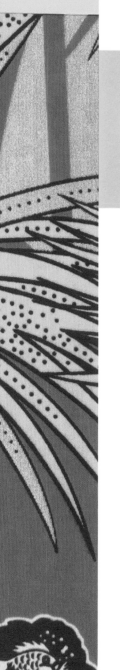

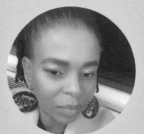

DREAMS, AMBITIONS AND A DIAGNOSIS OF HIV

Neo Moepi

I was a young adult, ambitious and looking forward to my education so that I would be better placed to look after myself. I wanted to be a television presenter. However, an opportunity came for me to come and work in the UK while I studied. My plan, upon my arrival in the UK, was to study Hotel Management and Hospitality. Six months down the line, I received the devastating news that I had tested positive to HIV, and this news affected my plans and mental health.

When I was diagnosed, I didn't know much about HIV. My recollection, with regards to anything to do with AIDS, was that things were really bad. There was so much to be scared about out there. People were dying, so I knew about a deadly disease called AIDS. I first heard about HIV when I was still a child. It didn't mean anything much to me at the time, but there was a big taboo about the illness and stereotypes that it affected gay men and women who were prostitutes.

Reflecting on my diagnosis and the events that followed

On reflection I am grateful that I received my diagnosis when I was here in the UK where support and treatment are so advanced and accessible to all. Although ART was new and still in development, at least I thought there was hope for me. The referral for peer support saved my life. It was through peer support that I realised I could start to live my life. Meeting women who had been living with HIV for 10 to 20 years, sharing testimonies that they were given six months to live, but they lived beyond, I will always have this in my mind. When I reflect, I also think that had I remained in Africa I probably would not be in this world today.

After I received my diagnosis, I felt the need to be part of the movement to change negative stereotypes, discrimination and stigma against people living with HIV. Through peer support I was able to achieve work in the sector where people living with HIV could thrive and live meaningful lives. The work that I have been involved in has helped to turn my life around and think positively when coming to terms with my diagnosis. As a result of this new perspective, I was able to obtain a university degree and have children.

One of the lowest points in my HIV journey was being diagnosed as diabetic after starting HIV treatment. I still struggle sometimes and blame myself for starting treatment, which is meant to help lower the viral load in my blood but has led to developing another condition.

Combating stigma in African communities

I started as a participant in the HIV sector, getting involved not only to get support for myself, but also to educate myself about living positively with HIV. Once I felt comfortable, I got involved in projects aimed at combating the stigma associated with HIV, especially within African communities. I volunteered my time to support others, but also spoke publicly about issues affecting us as Africans, challenging and voicing about policies made for us without us.

I feel African communities should come forward to be included from the beginning to the end, especially with research and access. There are a lot of obstacles for African communities, such as migration, cultural beliefs, shame and internalised stigma, which need to continue to be addressed. Allies can support, but as Africans we also have to show our faces and fight for our rights.

During my journey I have built positive relationships with other women living with HIV, building a lifelong network of support, both personally and professionally. This holds great meaning for me, because I do not have to pretend. I am able to be myself as a woman living with HIV.

Live life each day, as you do not know what tomorrow will bring.

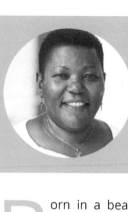

BENT, NOT BROKEN: LIVING POSITIVELY AND DYING WITH DIGNITY

Noerine Kaleeba

Born in a beautiful remote rural village, within a polygamous family of one father, four mothers and a cumulative total of 28 siblings, my childhood was surrounded by a happy hardworking environment. Top of the list of the many gifts my siblings and I received from our parents was the gift of access to formal education.

After completing my O-level education at Mount St Mary's High School, Namagunga, I enrolled on a three-year diploma training in Physiotherapy, becoming one of the first six Ugandan-trained physiotherapists. Up until then, all physiotherapists were being trained in Britain. We had a nine-month stint in the UK at the Robert Jones & Agnes Hunt Orthopaedic Hospital, Oswestry, before completing the diploma at Makerere University, Uganda. It was during this period of my stay in the UK that I met and made some lifelong friends who have remained key pillars of my resilience. I took interest and specialised in orthopaedics and children living with disabilities. I worked as the Director of the Cheshire Home for the Disabled and the School of Physiotherapy in Uganda, concurrently, for a number of years.

I got married in 1975 to my husband Christopher Kaleeba, a radiographer. We were blessed with four beautiful biological children, all of who are now fully grown professional women; three are parents themselves. Over the decades during which HIV has ravaged my family, I have been parent and sole provider for a large number of children, all of who are now adults with diverse professional skills, thanks to financial support given by my international network of Friends of Noerine Kaleeba (FONK).

In July 1983, my husband was run over by a bus. One of his legs was nearly severed and he needed a blood transfusion. Many friends and acquaintances supported us during this time. Finally, Chris was given eight pints of blood, donated by different people, which saved his life. At that time, blood was not screened for HIV in Uganda.

Unfortunately, Chris's life was never the same again. He used to complain of various pains in his body and a lack of energy, but we didn't think too much of it and put it down to the accident and his frustration about the life he felt he lost before the accident. Using my physiotherapy skills, I contributed to nursing him back to health. In April 1985, he was offered a scholarship through the British Council to study for a Masters in Education in Sociology and Business Administration in the UK. He left Uganda in May 1985 and enrolled at Hull University.

In June 1986, I received a call from the British Council informing me that Chris was gravely ill and had been admitted at Castle Hill Hospital in Hull. He had been found unconscious with a suspected case of cryptococcal meningitis. I had to contact a friend of mine who was a microbiologist to find out what that condition was. My friend responded by asking me to find out if my husband had been offered an HIV test. I asked about the AIDS test on my next call with the British Council representative and they told me that the AIDS test had come back positive.

The enormity of the positive HIV test did not register at the time, because everything was happening so fast. I was working two jobs and looking after four young children, but worse was still to come. I was told in that same phone call that the doctors didn't think my husband had long to live and they wanted me to travel to the UK as soon as possible.

Travel arrangements were made in five days with the help of the British Council, but it seemed like eternity, especially with my husband's health on a knife edge. I also had to make arrangements for my children to be taken care of at home and to make sure they attended school. One of my sisters volunteered to take on this huge responsibility.

When he was conscious, Chris recognised me. He was very ill and looked like a shadow of his old self, but I could not let on how shocked I was. At the hospital, the doctors and nurses let me know that we were the only black heterosexual couple they had ever had in relation to AIDS. I was counselled and offered an HIV test, which turned out to be negative. The negative results did not have any impact on me at the time partly, because I was circled with misery from seeing Chris in that condition.

Denial, fear, mystery, stigma and conspiracy theories

In September 1986, I left Chris in the hospital in Hull and returned to Uganda because my father was unwell. My father died the day before I arrived home, which was so painful for me, but I was also very aware that I might never see Chris alive again. It was a tough period in my life.

In Uganda, the AIDS issue had suddenly come to the forefront of the media and hospital discussions. At the same time, even with the increasing number of people being diagnosed with AIDS, there was denial, fear, mystery, stigma and conspiracy theories. I had made a point to be open about Chris's HIV diagnosis, because as a family we felt we had nothing to hide. We experienced a lot of stigma and discrimination from all walks of life, including and especially in the healthcare sector in Uganda. When I returned to work, some colleagues distanced themselves. I also noticed the anxiety in the faces of some neighbours whenever my family and I bumped into them. It was a challenging time. The AIDS awareness campaigns were inadequate, especially in an environment where there was no treatment, just a lot of death.

In October 1986, Chris decided that he wanted to leave the UK to return to Uganda, to become the face of AIDS. He was determined to raise awareness about the condition and help to reduce the stigma attached to it. Two days before his departure, he was discharged and allowed some respite at the London Lighthouse. He had been getting support from the Terrence Higgins Trust (THT) through its buddy system while at Castle Hill Hospital.

From Entebbe airport, although Chris was able to walk off the plane on his own, he was taken to Mulago Hospital in Kampala by ambulance. The ambulance was organised by the Welfare Officer from the British Council. Chris's stay at the hospital was to enable us to sort out things at home to make him comfortable. He was terrified of passing the virus on to his family, especially his children, even though with the little we knew of AIDS at the time that was unlikely.

At the time there were no antiretroviral medicines. Even drugs for opportunistic infections were in very short supply, partly due to the chronic shortages of all medicines, but more due to the negative attitude and apathy towards AIDS care within the entire healthcare system. Chris arrived back home with various types of palliative care medication generously donated by Castle Hill Hospital, which helped him for a few months before his final collapse and which we shared among the first few patients we were able to reach.

Growing HIV peer support: from the ground up

When Chris was finally able to come home it was not easy. I still had to work to bring in money, because now the whole family depended on my sole income; but I also had to make sure that my husband was being taken care of at home and my children were going to school. One of my sisters really helped me out a lot.

Chris's biggest challenge was his appetite. He couldn't keep any food down and was always vomiting. We used a lot of mixed herbal concoctions, mixed with different 'European medications' to enable him to eat and boost his energy. It was also during this period that Chris and I began talking about helping others who were being diagnosed as HIV positive. There was nothing being offered except to wait for people to die after being isolated, ostracised and stigmatised, and dying in so much pain because there was no HIV treatment.

While I was away at work, Chris would hold small group meetings with recently diagnosed people to exchange ideas and to support each other. He used his experience at Castle Hill Hospital and interaction with the buddy system at the THT and became a great resource to people who had lost all hope. The conversations my husband and I had, plus the small groups meetings, gave birth to The Aids Support Organisation (TASO), Uganda.

Chris didn't survive though. He got a final attack of cryptococcal meningitis and died in agonising pain on 23rd January 1987, at Mulago Hospital, Uganda's main and biggest hospital. The experience with the hospital staff at the time was uncomfortable and distressing. We were not treated with compassion as the fears and prejudices of the healthcare staff got the better of them. Even though I had anticipated my husband's death, I was not emotionally prepared for it. He died in undignified pain and suffering. Throughout the funeral period, I mourned for the loss of my husband, my orphaned children and so much more.

Life was never going to be the same: memories of compassion and care

After Chris died I had to pick myself up and get on with life, if only for my children. It became clear to me very quickly that life was never going to go back to the way it was before my husband's death. Memories of the compassion and tender loving care given to Chris at Castle Hill Hospital, contrasted with the negative experience of stigma and indifference we got at Mulago, propelled me to reach out and concentrate on supporting people living with AIDS. I couldn't just go back to work the way I did before; I had to do something different.

After the funeral, I mobilised the people who had previously met with Chris and we formed a support group. This group was joined by a few of my close friends, two of whom were physiotherapist, one nurse, one educationalist, and Dr Elly Katabira who had just set up the first AIDS specialised clinic in Mulago Hospital. This support group, though volatile due to the fact that the majority of members had AIDS and died within the first six months of our getting together, was the firm foundation upon which TASO Uganda was built. We adopted a unique theme of 'Living Positively and dying with dignity', which propelled us forward in these difficult days during which we lost friends, but also became the beacon of hope for increasing numbers of people who were getting diagnosed with AIDS.

Although I had tested HIV negative in the UK, I did not believe the results. I chose to live as though I was HIV positive; after all, most people who had heard about my husband's diagnosis and death took it for granted that it was a matter of time before I succumbed to AIDS. The doctor who had delivered my results in the UK was not sure why I was HIV negative.

Living positively

Under my leadership, TASO developed into a spontaneous self-help group that came out of the need for people living with HIV and AIDS wanting to blow off steam, cry, pray together and give each other hope. Most of the general information and country campaigns at that time focused on primary prevention. It was as if once a person was diagnosed with AIDS (with or without an HIV test), the only route was a painful death. We realised, however, that more of the people we were reaching with counselling and accurate information about positive living, were living longer and better-quality lives, even without HIV-specific treatment. We developed and promoted a Positive Living Package that has remained viable throughout the entire evolution of HIV prevention, treatment and care.

TASO was dependent on the voluntary participation of men and women living with HIV. In the beginning, we got most of our information from THT in the UK. We offered food, medicine, transport to hospital and other support that many struggling people living with HIV were desperate for. Unable to cope with the huge demand and minimal donations at TASO, we approached the Director of the AIDS Control Programme in Uganda at the time. Even though he had not completely bought into the TASO idea, we were endorsed and received the first one-off initial funding for the self-help group. ActionAid Uganda was the first internationally linked organisation to provide technical and financial support to TASO. TASO was able to get funding for the services of a physician, as well as financial support for me and the doctor to obtain training in HIV counselling in the UK. This leap of faith by ActionAid proved and influenced other partners like USAID to provide increasing technical and financial support to TASO from very early on, until today where TASO continues to enjoy a very positive relationship with diverse international partners.

TASO was formally established in 1987 by 16 volunteers (12 of them HIV positive). We focused on breaking the silence on stigma, igniting the passion of families and communities to care and support each other. We also wanted to support and strengthen people living with AIDS to live their lives with dignity and give a positive and human face to AIDS.

Within the first year of our journey, all the 12 HIV positive founder members died, but within that same period we registered 850 people.

Over 35 years on, TASO is considered a model of best practice. It continues to evolve and to be replicated in various forms outside of Uganda. It provides counselling training, social support, clinical care, support for orphans and vulnerable children and much more. TASO broke the taboo by talking about sex, death, inheritance and traditional laws that impact negatively on women and children. It is also the second recipient of the Global Fund to Fight HIV, TB and Malaria in Uganda, a role TASO has performed.

Influencing policy and strengthening the global movement

Through my frontline work, starting and developing TASO, I was able to access many international opportunities, including speaking at conferences and serving on global AIDS commissions and boards of many HIV organisations. In 1995 I was recruited to join Professor Peter Piot, a microbiologist researcher, and became a staff member of the small team that set up the foundation upon which UNAIDS stands today. I served in the role of Partnership and Community Mobilisation Advisor for ten years until 2006, when I took voluntary retirement.

This move to Geneva into a global UNAIDS role provided me with numerous opportunities to influence policy and strengthen community responses to health and development challenges. It provided me and TASO with the opportunity to detach, without abandoning the cause, enabling current TASO leadership to innovate and grow the organisation without being smothered by the founder. The TASO family graciously gave me a role as Patron and Founder, which is largely advisory and ceremonial.

This move to global level also enabled my children to access international education and obtain a global perspective to the life with which they now face in their diverse careers and parenting roles.

As Chair of the Founding Board of ActionAid International and later as member and vice-chair of AMREF Africa Health Board, and more recently as a member of the VSO international Board I have provided opportunities for community voices to influence policy on health and development. I have also earned global and national recognition, from the King of Buganda, The Uganda Golden Jubilee Medal from Uganda government and three Honorary doctorates, one from each of Nkumba University, Uganda, Dundee University, Scotland, and Geneva School of Diplomacy and International Relations, Switzerland.

In my retirement, I am as committed as ever to carrying on providing guidance and advice on the issues that have challenged, but also served so often to strengthen, my resilience across my lifetime.

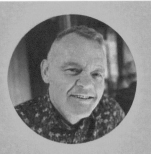

I KNEW I WAS DIFFERENT, JUST DIDN'T KNOW WHAT IT WAS CALLED: 'YOUNG MAN ARE YOU A HOMOSEXUAL?'

Shaun Mellors

Life growing up

I grew up in a very sheltered and poor environment during apartheid in South Africa. My family were very conservative and religious, and I remember that we moved house constantly. Even though I grew up poor and in a complex and toxic family structure, I only realised and appreciated my privilege many years later. My father was the only breadwinner – very common in white South Africa for the husband to work, whilst the mother 'plays the housewife'. I never knew whether this was by choice or unspoken agreement. I was the middle child of three, all boys. An additional son came along in 1984.

We lived mostly in areas where my father could find a job, and this meant that we would often move to the far-flung corners of what was then called Transvaal. We were not close as a family and I don't recall any meaningful conversations about the 'birds and the bees', relationships, sexuality or love. When I started high school, I was sent to boarding school, following in the footsteps of my elder brother. Boarding school was in many ways a godsend, as I was able to experience a bit more freedom and escape from the difficulties at home.

I knew at a young age that I was different, but I did not know what to call it – I did not have a label for it. I remember driving in the car one day with my parents. I was sitting in the back and we stopped at a traffic light. We saw an effeminate man cross the road with another man and I said to my parents, 'Look at that man!' (obviously identifying with

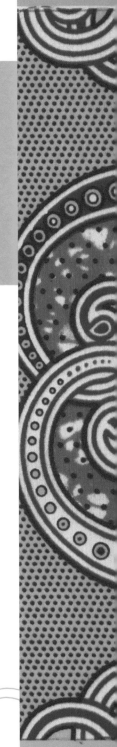

something in him). My parent's response was, 'Don't look at him, he is sick and needs help!' I was left flabbergasted, as this must mean that I am sick and that I, too, needed help.

As long as I can remember I have wanted to become a teacher. It was what I dreamed of. I had a girlfriend in my final years of high school and we both wanted to become teachers and we both had the white-picket fence and two-and-a-half children dream. I planned for this since the start of high school and applied to go to teacher training college at the Johannesburg College of Education affiliated to the University of Witwatersrand. I was accepted (she unfortunately was not), but I was ill-prepared for what was to come. I was not worldly wise, did not have the life skills required to navigate my newfound freedoms and I was not ready for the big city life and all that it had to offer.

Exploring life's possibilities

I was a young, confused man in the big city probably for the first time in his life. I was amazed by the lights, the options, the freedoms that living in the big city offered. I was free to explore the uncertainty of what I was feeling about who and what I was – and boy did I explore. I remember the fear and excitement of going into a gay bar for the first time in my life, challenged by what this was saying about me, uncertain if this was what I wanted; the exhilaration of having sex with another man for the first time and the immense shame that I felt afterwards; how easily I was able to 'fall in love' and declare my love, but also how easily I fell out of love. I was not able to share any of this with anyone in my family or my circle of friends. I even had a few girlfriends at college. I was ashamed because so much of what I felt and thought about myself was considered a sin by my family, by community and my faith. I was 'sick and needed help'.

Halfway through my first year at uni, I was called up to do my compulsory two-year national army service. I dreaded this experience and when I eventually arrived at base camp, I told them that I was at college and studying to become a teacher. The request fell on deaf ears. I did not agree with what was happening, the two-year national conscription and did not want to fight in their war. I eventually found the courage to tell the army that I was a homosexual and was given a dishonourable discharge six months later, as gay men and women could not serve in the army. I was relieved. My parents were disappointed.

This meant that I had to repeat my first year at uni, only this time I was better prepared. I explored my sexuality with a new sense of acceptance and tried to balance study with living life. In December 1986, I was working at a supermarket and collapsed one day at work. I thought it was related to exams, poor eating and general exhaustion from trying to balance life. I was rushed to what was then called the Johannesburg General Hospital. In casualty a doctor examined me and found swollen glands, asked about weight loss, mentioned something about thrush and asked me, 'Young man, are you a homosexual?'

I stuttered and stammered and said 'Y-yes, doctor.' She drew back the curtain and went to speak to some colleagues appearing a few minutes later with a very serious look on her face. She looked at me over her glasses and said, 'Young man, I am sorry to tell you this, but I think that you have AIDS and about six months left to live.'

I remember looking up at the clock. It was 16:10 and it was 24th December.

When I was diagnosed, the landscape was shaped by fear and ignorance, understandably so in those early years. Many in South Africa at that time still thought that HIV was an American disease. There was little understanding of the difference between HIV and AIDS, very few clinics offering support and no support groups or organisations of people living with HIV. In many ways, AIDS was seen as the broom that would sweep society 'clean'. The first reported cases in South Africa were initially among gay men – the misfits, the sinners, those who were beyond help. This narrative was also emphasised in the media, whilst HIV largely went unnoticed in the broader society.

In many ways, the early days of activism and peer support was my treatment. We had the opportunity to shape and define a patient response, and I think in many ways a response that has led the way for other diseases, too.

Lack of choices: the need to regain control

I had no choice really. I was not able to go back to teacher training college as I was told, 'An AIDS victim will never be able to teach,' and that I should 'enjoy the time that you have left'. I believed it! I was lost, confused, isolated. What was I going to do with the remaining six months that I had left? How do I tell my parents? I found a casual job to earn some income and waited for the moment to come. Six months came and went, and I was still very much alive. I had not developed those purple blotches and did not end up with pneumonia. The six months soon turned to a year, and I was still very much alive. It was then that I had a mind-shift – perhaps I can live with this virus, but for me to do that, I need to control it and not allow it to control me.

I was seen at the HIV clinic at the Johannesburg General, and I started an informal support group. We would meet at a friend's flat in Hillbrow, arrange tea and biscuits and meet on a fortnightly basis. It was so comforting to be meeting with other people living with HIV, but it was also quite scary, as many of those acquaintances and friends became ill. However, this also became the focus and how we were portrayed in the media – and this was definitely not a positive image to those of us living with HIV or to those family members. Whilst I recognised some of these images, I did not recognise myself and many of my friends. I was not a victim or a patient. I was not sick, thin, frail or dying. I wanted to change the image and portrayal of people living with HIV and that is what led to me going public about my HIV status in the late 1980s.

After that, in many ways HIV became my career as I started in working with and for HIV-related organisations in South Africa, speaking at conferences and advocating for the rights of people living with HIV. I was passionate about the work, though initially it did not feel like work. It was more like a drive, a purpose, a commitment – something that had to be done.

I have had a blessed life, much of it shaped and informed by my experiences of living with HIV and coming to terms with my sexuality.

Reflecting on living with HIV: empowerment

One of my highlights was starting the first support groups for people living with HIV, meeting in different people's homes for tea, support and solidarity: those moments of sharing insights of dealing with thrush, or what to do about disclosure, or celebrating the life of another friend lost.

Another of my highlights was attending my first international conference for people living with HIV and AIDS in London in September 1991. This was organised by the International Steering Committee of People Living with HIV and AIDS run by the impressive Dietmar Bolle. This was my empowerment conference, as it was my first time sitting in a room with so many different, diverse, complex and beautiful people living with HIV. I met many of my heroes at this conference and also established many long-term friendships – and yes, also fell in love!

A significant event in my life came in 1992 when I shared a platform with Nelson Mandela at the first National AIDS Convention of South Africa (NACOSA). I had the privilege of speaking immediately after him at this important meeting that was the starting point for the development of the first post-apartheid national AIDS strategy.

This then led in 1994 to working at the AIDS Consortium at Wits University with Edwin Cameron and supporting the development of the National AIDS Charter on Rights and Responsibilities. In the same year I co-founded the National Association of People Living with HIV and AIDS South Africa.

A personal highlight and significant historical event occurred in 1994, when I represented South Africa at the Gay Olympics in New York City. It was the first time that South Africa was invited back into the Gay Games Federation post-apartheid. It was an incredible and very emotional experience, which led to my being selected as one of the outstanding South Africans to carry the 2004 Athens Olympic Torch as it went through South Africa together with the lovely Prudence Mabele, a South African activist for the rights of women and children living with HIV.

I was one of the first people living with HIV to lead the Global Network of People Living with HIV as its coordinator from 1995 to 1998. These were joyous, exciting, intense years. Developing, what is now GNP+ from a tiny loft office in Amsterdam, with one other staff member (and a committed board), was an incredible honour and such a privilege. It was also incredibly political and exhausting.

I also helped to organise and chair the 7th International Conference for People Living with HIV and AIDS in Cape Town, South Africa (6th–10th March 1995) on behalf of GNP+ and the International Community of Women Living with HIV and AIDS (ICW).

My other contributions to the HIV sector

I contributed to the development of the Greater Involvement of People Living with HIV and AIDS (GIPA) principle during the 1994 Paris AIDS Summit. I have also represented people living with HIV in various platforms and capacities:

- Co-chairing the international task team to end HIV restrictions related to travel, stay and residence with UNAIDS
- Board member for the communities living with and affected by HIV, TB and malaria delegation to the Global Fund Board

- Chairing the Global Fund Partnership Forum and co-chairing the Global Fund Strategy and Impact Committee

Being in the spotlight: the highs and the lows

The lows were very much related to some of the highlights, as sometimes an issue started off as a low-light, but soon turned into a positive and sometimes even a highlight – for instance, the discrimination that I experienced as a person living with HIV and being public about it. I lost a job in the hotel industry but took legal action. I was denied entry into several countries (USA, Canada, Singapore, China) because of my public HIV status, but fought against these restrictions through the help of many organisations and colleagues.

One of the most significant low-lights has been the enormous sense of loss and wasted opportunity of friends who died far too soon. I have realised that dealing with death in my 20s is very different from dealing with death in my 50s. Many of my friends (and lovers) who died when I was in my 20s are people whom I had intense, beautiful and meaningful relationships with – but they were short, as I met most of them in my 20s. However, losing friends now is more difficult as there has been a journey of 30 or more years travelled, often through difficult and dark times, but also joyous and fun things. We managed to experience and live life, so in some ways it is as if chapters of my book of life are closing, and I miss them enormously.

I commemorated my 35th year of living with HIV on 24th December 2021. It was a reflective day, as they always are. I have not always enjoyed Christmas and avoided too many festivities because of this anniversary, but I realised that I am only spiting myself by allowing HIV to control what should be an important celebration of family, faith and friends. I decided to change my outlook and had a very special Christmas with family. I still don't like the commercialisation of Christmas and the pressure of buying gifts, but as I enter the autumn of my life, I want to apply the lessons that I have learnt, appreciate the gift of ageing, and ensure that I enjoy life to the full.

Doing life together: relationships with most meaning for me

Most of those relationships have been long-term friendships. Many of those friends are no longer on this place called earth, but still very much in my heart: friends who experienced doing life together; experienced the ups and downs; carrying and being carried; crying and supporting. They were friendships where we were trudging along the frontlines of the HIV response, where we witnessed and experienced things that shaped the rest of our lives, and friendships where there was no judgement but rather acceptance – or at least a willingness to learn and understand.

What I value most about these relationships is being able to have open, honest and direct conversations that have been enormously helpful and continue to be. Yes, they are difficult to initiate or to hear, but if the words are spoken and received with the right intent, it can only make us grow.

I have learnt never to judge a book by its cover and that there is always lots of interesting information and insights in those chapters and in between the lines. I just need to make the effort to read it.

One of the most important things – no, critical things – is how the role of community has been emphasised repeatedly in the HIV response. Ensuring that those living with the disease are integrally involved in decisions that impact our lives from policy to programming, implementation to evaluation and that communities have resources (financial, technical and capacity) to fulfil these important roles is a non-negotiable. We need to recognise community experience and community leadership for the expertise that it is.

It is sometimes hard to grasp that I have been living with HIV for longer than I lived without HIV, and that I have been on ARV treatment for 26 out of the 35 years. When I used to do public speaking about living with HIV, I was always asked what my secret for living with HIV so long was.

I don't have a secret. I think it has been a combination of things – a lucky roll of the dice, genetic make-up and a resilient approach and positive mindset, to name but a few. I try and apply the sensible things in my life like healthy eating, regular exercise and doing things that I enjoy. I have found that exercise is so important not only to keep me grounded, but also because it's good for my mental health. This is probably the most important investment that we can make in ourselves: looking after our physical and mental health.

Acceptance is giving up hope of a different past.

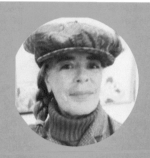

THE RISE OF THE FEMININE POWER: THE BEAUTY AND ENERGY OF AFRICAN CULTURES

Silvia Petretti

was born in Rome, Italy. I came to London in 1987 after my mum died. I loved this city and the richness of cultures. I studied African Arts and Languages at SOAS and spent most of my 20s travelling in West Africa, especially in Nigeria, where I researched textiles, and then got involved in writing a film on the legendary musician Fela Anikulapo Kuti.

I went back to Rome for a few years in 1992 and set up an organisation to promote African dance and music with a group of Italian women. We were called Kanyelang. In Italy we were just starting to see more migrants from Africa, and we wanted Italians to see the beauty and energy of African cultures. We were organising workshops with teachers from all over Africa and the Caribbean. We even organised a trip to Senegal with over 20 people to study drumming and dance.

I was diagnosed with HIV in 1997, in Rome. That was the worst year of my life. My grandmother, who I had grown up with, was very sick and died, my father had dementia, and I did not have a job or much support around me. I was a carer for my nan and dad. I spent six months crying, full of fear and shame. I never felt so lonely, but soon I decided that if I was going to die, I'd better do something useful with the time I had left.

In 1999, I moved back to London to do a MSc in Development Studies and was referred to Positively Women by my HIV doctor. I immediately loved the organisation and the ethos of peer support. All the staff were also women living with HIV. I started volunteering, and when a job became available I became a member of staff. Most of the women at Positively Women at that time were African, and I felt very at home.

I was really down after my diagnosis and thought I did not have long to live. The women I met at Positively Women showed me that you could still have a life with HIV. HIV did not need to be a barrier to a good life. You could still have love, sex, fun, look good, dress up and go clubbing. I became quickly very passionate about activism and that other women should have support and information, a safe space to process the HIV diagnosis. I did not want for any woman to ever feel so lonely and ashamed as I felt when I was diagnosed. Positively Women had a beautiful building, with a lot of space. We had two support groups a week, with a hot meal. It felt like a home, like a place where people cared about us. So many of us were not from the UK and we did not have our families here. Positively Women was our family.

Managing the uncertainty and learning to see a future: finding a voice to silence stigma

When I was first diagnosed, HIV treatments were new. Initially I was on 18 pills a day, some with food, some without food, with horrible side effects. Stigma was massive and telling a potential partner that you were living with HIV was really terrifying, because there was no U=U, and you had to use condoms religiously. The medications were new, and we did not know how/if they would have worked long term. Everything felt really uncertain and it was difficult to imagine the future. However, there was a lot of support.

My greatest high was deciding to be open about my HIV status in 2004. I was so fed up with the stigma. It became clear to me that if I wanted a world without stigma I had to create it. I had to fight for it. Being open was about telling the world that I was not ashamed, that I had nothing to hide. My motto is 'Stigma will end when people with HIV are visible and heard.' My first big public thing was to pose for a sculpture made by the artist Marc Quinn. It was a cast of my body made with my HIV medications and a special wax. The sculpture was at the entrance of the Wellcome Trust Gallery on Euston Road for many years. It was very beautiful and incredibly empowering.

I always had a great affinity with African cultures because of my studies and travel. I had a lot of support from African women at Positively Women, especially Angelina Namiba, Beatrice Naubilya, Winnie Sseruma, Memory Sachikonye. Those were the first women I saw speaking up and being activists. I would not be where I am today without their inspiration, support, encouragement and humour.

I hope people will remember me as someone who cared about others, who tried to make things a little better, even if I made mistakes. I have not been afraid to speak my truth, even when it is difficult and against the grain. Often women with HIV are forgotten, or just an afterthought, in a world that is still mainly run by men. I would like to remind people that they need to listen to us, as women.

We are here to share power and create change.

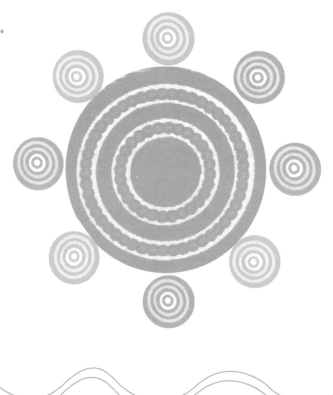

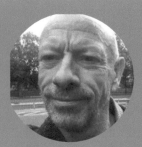

THE ART OF WRITING ABOUT HIV: CAMPAIGNING FOR SOCIAL CHANGE

Simon Collins

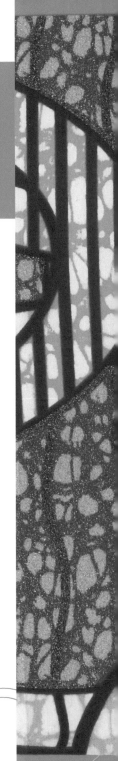

am an HIV positive gay man, born in London where I have lived most of my life.

I have been living with HIV for over 30 years and spent a lot of this time tracking HIV research. In April 2000, I was one of the people who founded HIV i-Base, where I still work. I am also interested in supporting community networks, especially with links to research.

Although I write about HIV treatment, I only really learnt about science later in life. I was mainly interested in art subjects at school and I wasn't particularly academic. Punk music was just breaking and I saw plenty of live bands, including getting to Rock Against Racism in Victoria Park. I also liked social history.

When I left school, I went to art college. Courses were still free and I don't think I would have gone otherwise. Although I wasn't a very good artist, I started reading everything I could, visited every exhibition, saw every fringe film, and became more socially, politically and sexually aware.

From one perspective, the 1980s was a very dynamic and lively time. I came out as a gay man, lived with my first boyfriend in a flat in Haringey, and quickly became interested in lesbian and gay rights. I also met people who were fighting for other progressive social changes, for example, working on campaigns that were anti-racist and anti-apartheid, and supporting the women's and labour movements.

From 1985 to 1989 I worked at a community printshop called CopyArt, which ran from a squat in Camden. One shop was behind King's Cross station roughly half-way between the Scala Cinema and the Mutoid Waste Company. We provided cheap printing and access to the photocopiers, supporting hundreds of community organisations and social campaigns and a wide range of artists, poets and other performers. Nightclubs and DJs designed and printed flyers, and people organising marches could come to print placards.

I became involved in various social and left-wing political groups. This included supporting London Labour councils that were developing progressive policies on lesbian and gay rights. Sometimes I went on TV or radio or spoke at local schools. I was active in support groups for the miners', printworkers' and seafarer strikes. I helped organise several marches and demonstrations, including the London march against Section 28 that banned talking about being gay in schools.

Mainstream life in the UK was still very sexist, racist and homophobic especially throughout national TV and newspaper; try looking at cartoons printed in The Sun at the time. Social divisions were made worse by a Conservative government that was increasingly right wing, wanting to dismantle the welfare state and break the Labour movement. This government supported apartheid in South Africa and Pinochet in Chile. Everything collectively owned by the country was steadily sold to private companies: water, gas, electricity, railways, airports, social housing, etc. The profits supported tax cuts for people who generally voted Conservative. Wealthy people became richer and more than four million people were unemployed.

I learnt about HIV from the free weekly paper Capital Gay, and went to the early public meeting of the Terrence Higgins Trust (THT) at Conway Hall, but I didn't get involved in the earliest HIV activism. I was supportive, of course, and active in other ways, because I remember flyposting 'FUND AIDS RESEARCH' across the tombstone billboard adverts in Waterloo – but I don't think many people noticed.

This political context is important, because the Conservative government has a terrible history where HIV is concerned. Rather than a medical or scientific response, it used HIV to promote a socially divisive agenda based on so-called family values. Rather than working with the communities and organisations that were most severely affected, they launched a national campaign on billboards and TV that primarily scared young people from having sex. The leaflet they sent to every household divided people into us and them (and people living with HIV were 'them').

The government response laid a foundation for the decades of fear and discrimination against people living with HIV that we are still trying to overcome today. At exactly the time when sexual health should have been included in schools, it was blocked by Section 28. Laws were passed that attacked the rights of lesbians and gay men, reinforced discrimination, and led to tens of thousands of young gay men becoming HIV positive.

Although I knew about HIV, it remained in the next room for a long time

Other than the concerns about trying to stay safe, HIV didn't directly affect me until 1987. This sounds terrible to say because I knew about HIV and AIDS, but it was still at a distance, in the room next door. Then in February 1987, the activist Mark Ashton died, after only being in hospital for about ten days. I was lucky to know Mark and his death had a huge impact that changed me. At 26, he was about a year older than me. That was way too young. It is difficult to think back to those times. It doesn't really make sense that I am now 61.

Then, in October the same year, my partner Nick was told that he was HIV positive, after being tested without his consent. Steadily, over the next year or two, at least half of a network of maybe 100 close friends also tested positive.

HIV affected everything, even when just trying to carry on with regular life. I spent less time on demonstrations and more time on my personal life and friends. I left my job to work from home instead, although I still probably worked too much. For all the fear about HIV, I was lucky to know other people going through the same things. HIV created strong friendships, but could also be very isolating, as even gay venues were not particularly welcoming if you became more ill.

One way to cope with HIV was to lead a healthier lifestyle, to manage infections as they occurred and to keep up-to-date with news about treatment. I also attended too many funerals. Even though Nick was becoming more ill, we always believed that living a day at a time until there was effective treatment would be OK. A Pet Shop Boys song has a line: 'I always thought that you'd be here with me.' It is true; I believed Nick would make it and I hoped everyone else would, too. Of course, I was wrong.

Nick died in 1994 when he was only 36 – and he really wanted to be 40. He fought really hard. By this time, my CD4 count was only 60 and it steadily dropped to single figures over the next year. I used AZT for a short time, then DDI when it involved dissolving large white tablets in water, and lamivudine on open access, but only for maybe a month at a time and without much effect. I continued working, but managing HIV was now full time, even living one day at a time. By 1996 I had become pretty ill. I developed gut infections such as microsporidia and cryptosporidium. (Morphine helped with chronic diarrhoea and maybe my mood.) I had fungal infections that made it difficult to eat. I had CMV in both eyes. (I learnt the eye chart so I could keep my driving licence.) My weight dropped to 45kg. When I spent time at the Chelsea and Westminster Hospital, friends were often on the same ward. Luckily, some of them also survived.

Then, without any expectations, I started combination antiretroviral therapy (ART, then called HAART) and I started to get better. My weight and energy levels increased every week, many opportunistic infections resolved and over the first year my CD4 count steadily increased to about 100.

In about mid-1996, I saw an advert for a new HIV organisation called AIDS Treatment Project (ATP). I was still too ill to get to the first meeting, but I went to the second and immediately started to volunteer. ATP was focused on HIV treatment and because I knew it worked, I wanted to become actively involved.

ATP had two main projects. The first was to publish a technical review of the latest research advances called DrFax. As the name suggests, this was sent by fax to doctors, and this was done every two weeks because information was changing so fast. This was an activist strategy to make sure our doctors were up to date.

The second was to run a treatment information phoneline. Anyone could ask about HIV treatment, but most of the calls were about the new drugs. People just wanted to know whether they worked and if any side effects would be OK.

Both these services are still running. DrFax became HIV Treatment Bulletin, probably making it one of the longest-running community HIV publications. HIV i-Base still runs a treatment phoneline, now expanded to an online service, that answers thousands of individual questions each year from all over the world.

Quack remedies, support groups and the era of HIV treatment

In 1996, the outlook for anyone living with HIV was still grim, especially if your CD4 count was dropping and you were already becoming ill. The first HIV drugs were not effective and this led to many people looking at alternative approaches. Some therapies, such as massage or acupuncture, could at least make you feel better. Others, like Chinese herbs were intolerable. None of these could increase my CD4 count and others were quack remedies with no evidence benefit and easy potential for harm.

The UK also had hundreds of HIV organisations that provided support in different ways. Some of the national organisations (THT, National AIDS Trust and the UK Coalition) had lobbied to make sure people living with HIV were able to access welfare benefits. Others provided support for housing, legal aid, meals (Food Chain), buddies (THT) and respite/ palliative care (including the London Lighthouse, Bethany in Cornwall and the Mildmay). People living with HIV also developed national and local support groups. These included Body Positive groups (in at least 30 UK cities and towns). It also included groups that met the specific needs of women (Positively Women), people who had become positive from injecting drugs (Mainliners) or from blood products (Birchgrove), and people from Black and Asian backgrounds (Blackliners). By 1996, there were probably about 100 African support groups.

ATP was largely a volunteer-based peer organisation and a majority of the people involved were living with HIV. This was very different from most other national HIV charities, which employed very few people who were openly HIV positive. While some of the best advocates I have known have been HIV negative, the culture of an organisation is very different if the people who it has been set up to help are also included and visible.

ATP also focused on treatment. A lot of us became involved because we had direct experience of both HIV and treatment. We ran workshops for people to learn more, with training from leading HIV doctors. If you contacted most HIV organisations in 1996 with a question about your treatment, you would be sent back to ask your doctor. ATP was different. If someone wanted information, we would research this and send it to them. We also said that people living with HIV should be able to make their own decisions about treatment, not just have these made for us.

The new treatments caught nearly everyone by surprise. The UK had developed expert HIV services including medical care, support, and social rights. However, some HIV doctors and most HIV organisations did not appreciate the importance of combination therapy and how it needed to be used, which was to include at least three active drugs, be strong enough to make viral load undetectable and have high levels of adherence.

If you missed any one of these, the combination would likely fail, and drug resistance would limit future options.

This meant ATP often provided information that was different from that of someone's doctor or even the first HIV guidelines. The experience of using evidence to look at different options has informed all of my work since.

DrFax was edited by the osteopath Paul Blanchard, who had waited for combination therapy rather than using single drugs, even though his CD4 was severely knocked and he had extensive Kaposi's sarcoma. He understood the principals of treatment and he made sure DrFax reported on the risk from drug resistance and cross-resistance, often before new drugs were even approved. This was at a time when many HIV organisations were more worried about possible side effects and when new UK guidelines still suggested that only two drugs might be OK.

Over the next couple of years, seven or eight new drugs were approved and others were in development. Some were definitely better than others and getting the choice right could make a big difference to your long-term health. However, drug manufacturers used large budgets to influence prescribing.

ATP provided information to update the way some clinics provided care and challenged other HIV charities that missed the urgency of getting treatment right. We were also a diverse group from different backgrounds, largely as volunteers. This is where I first met Paul Blanchard, Polly Clayden, Hope Mhereza, Winnie Sseruma, Simon Mwendapole, William Babumba, Badru Male, Henry Mumbi, Andrew Wilson-Jones and many others. I was lucky to get to learn with people who had very different experiences and this diversity has been essential in everything we tried to do since.

ATP rented office space from the UK Coalition of HIV Positive People, who also published Positive Nation. This magazine, under the guidance of Graham McKerrow as editor, actively supported and developed the diversity of HIV activists from African, gay men, heterosexual, people who used IV drugs and haemophilia communities, including as columnists and on the front covers. Thanks to Graham's encouragement. I wrote a Q&A column for Positive Nation and was supported to report from CROI in 1998.

Meeting activists from Europe and the USA also showed that we could go further than just asking our doctor about treatment. That other sources included talking to researchers and drug companies. That early study results were presented at conferences long before they were published in medical journals, and it was just as important to translate technical information into everyday language so other people living with HIV could follow new research.

Finding a new focus, connecting back to life and HIV activism

I was lucky to come to HIV work when the new treatments made this a time of hope. It meant that many friends survived.

Learning about treatment gave me a new focus and connected me back to life. I joined a new network of people who also wanted to give something back after returning to better health. I started out as a volunteer, then worked part time, and eventually full time.

I have met so many people who I wouldn't otherwise have met and some are now old friends. This also includes activists from other countries including with the Treatment Action Campaign in South Africa, who do amazing work in often much more difficult settings, and I was lucky to be able to link with a global network of activists working on better access to treatment.

In 1988, I went to my first World AIDS Conference on a community scholarship and for the first time saw some of the excesses and contradictions of the HIV response. Efavirenz was launched as a breakthrough drug and was lavishly marketed in five-star chateaux on the banks of Lake Geneva. However, the conference also made it clear that the new drugs were only for people living in high-income countries. Many of the other community delegates had no access to treatment when they returned home.

The most significant HIV achievement though was to see generic treatment steadily become available globally. Many people thought the early goal of getting three million people on ART by 2005 (the 3x5 campaign) would not be possible; but now more than 28 million people are on ART in low-income countries where most of the HIV positive people live. This didn't happen fast enough and is still not perfect, but it showed that social and political changes need to match any scientific breakthroughs.

Since then, treatment has become more effective, easier to take and with fewer side effects. In 1996, I used to take a handful of pills each day, with a complicated schedule and difficult side effects, but it kept me alive. There are now (in high-income countries) ten different single-pill combinations, plus a long-acting injectable treatment.

My personal lows come from friends who still died too young because HIV treatment didn't arrive in time or because of complications later. I have lost many friends, including Paul Blanchard and Paul Decle, who both helped set up HIV i-Base. Other activists who died too young include Antony Kwok, Alan Norburn, Martyn Flynn, Simon Mwendapole, Darren Ravenor, Andrew Mosane and Bea Wheeler. I would also include Elias Phiri who was not HIV positive, but who died from Covid-19 in 2021.

Building networks in difficult times

I have already mentioned important friends, because nothing related to HIV is done on your own. The first community activists worked in much more difficult times, and they built a network of services that informed everything that came afterwards.

Over the 25 years I have been involved in the HIV sector, I have met hundreds of researchers, usually activist doctors who take on second careers as researchers to make medical care better. They have supported community involvement, invested time, been incredibly patient and encouraged our involvement.

Polly Clayden who cofounded HIV i-Base after we left ATP, is largely responsible for the project surviving, and has become a leading expert on women's health, HIV and pregnancy, children's health, and global access to HIV meds.

HIV i-Base was lucky to have been given a start-up grant from the Monument Trust, which also supported us later when we were exhausted from running month-to-month for so many years. Without this support, HIV i-Base would not have been possible, so I would like to thank Stewart and his late partner Simon for trusting us. This is true for other supporters, too, whether individuals, charities or pharmaceutical companies – even when we are critical of their drugs or pricing policies.

Thanks to the NHS, I am personally lucky to have had great medical care from nurses and doctors, who have incredible skills and dedication. I don't think I would be here otherwise.

Key highlights from working within the sector

HIV i-Base developed a few projects that were not being done by others and we stuck with these. It is good to have kept these running.

I like the UK Community Advisory Board (UK-CAB). Loosely based on the European CAB, this was started by HIV i-Base, getting 25 UK activists in the same room to work collectively on treatment issues. This was at a time when HIV organisations were otherwise often competing for funding rather than collaborating. I like that the CAB has always represented the diversity of the UK epidemic, that anyone can join and that there are now more than 700 members. Run by an elected steering group, and thanks to many years of support from Memory Sachikonye, the UK-CAB is a great network.

I like that the phone line evolved into an international email and online Q&A service that has answered more than 100,000 questions about HIV treatment. I think i-Base is the only organisation that does this. We recently had an email about treatment from a woman in New Guinea who was diagnosed during pregnancy. I can't explain how we connect from our small office near Tower Bridge, but I like that we do.

Even though the need for printed booklets has changed as people get information in different ways, I like that HIV i-Base still produces resources that are free to NHS clinics. The latest version of Introduction to ART was the 24th edition.

As a result of the work we have done, research groups now actively include people living with HIV at all stages of trial design. I was very lucky to be involved in two very important studies that both ran for about ten years. The START study provided data to support universal access to ART and the PARTNER studies produced the main evidence to prove that effective treatment prevents HIV transmission.

I am happy if HIV i-Base is known by people living with HIV who need information about treatment, but otherwise it doesn't need to be a household name.

There are always more
things to be done, and more things
that can be done faster.

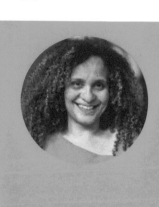

SEX IN THE SUBURBS: A DESIRE TO DO SOMETHING MORE MEANINGFUL WITH MY LIFE

Susan Cole-Haley

" The good news is you don't have syphilis. The bad news is you have HIV. Oh, and you have about seven years to live."

That's how I received my HIV diagnosis from a cheerily incompetent immigration doctor in the USA. I had just married my second husband (I've had three so far, I collect them like stamps) and it didn't cross my mind for a moment that the routine HIV test would come back positive. But there I was in rural Louisiana, far from home in London, essentially being told I wouldn't live to see my two children, who were five and seven at the time, grow to be men. This was 1998, so clearly the doctor was very wrong about my life expectancy, but the trauma of my diagnosis clung for years.

The period around my traumatic HIV diagnosis, living in a strange country away from family and friends, given a death sentence with two young children, in an unhappy relationship and being unable to work because of immigration constraints was probably my biggest personal low. I tasted the misery of an uncertain immigration status, needing my mother to send me money via Western Union to feed my children and at a time when I didn't know if I would live long enough to see them grow to be men. That was a shit time, but luckily it passed when I moved back home.

I was a teenager in the 1980s when the 'Don't Die of Ignorance' campaign about AIDS was launched in the UK, with harrowing TV adverts featuring tombstones and, inexplicably, icebergs. Alarming, yes: but something I thought would ever affect me? Absolutely not. It was something that happened to other people, not privately educated girls from suburban London. I went to university in Cardiff, buoyed by my self-perceived edgy coolness of being a DJ and on the Student Union executive. On Wales Today burning an effigy of Margaret Thatcher? Tick. Occupying buildings and marching against apartheid and student loans, convinced I would change the world? Tick. Getting married at 22 and having a baby at 23? OK, not so edgy, but I had married the President of the university drama society (ex-husband number one) who was meant to become a famous actor but worked in HR instead. And I had a stint working as a research psychologist before becoming knocked up with child number one (of four), who eventually went to Oxford University. I'm sorry, I'm a black mother, I had to find a way to get that boast in somewhere.

So, let's jump forward to 1998, divorced from husband number one, just married to husband number two (I've had handbags that have lasted longer than both those marriages), just diagnosed with HIV. Fortunately, I was diagnosed at a time when combination therapy had just become available, meaning that people with HIV could expect to live a long life. Yet the doctor who diagnosed me hadn't told me this. My mother, back in London took out a subscription to AIDS Treatment Update, a publication from NAM aidsmap, where I actually work today. That's where I got the information about the reality of HIV. Since then, knowledge about HIV has been the most empowering thing for me. I voraciously consumed all the information I could, and continue to do so today.

I returned to the UK two years later with my children (minus ex-husband number two) and began working in corporate sales in the City, determined that HIV wouldn't be a barrier to me making money and dressing my sons up in garish matchy-matchy designer outfits. That changed on 11th September 2001. I remember watching the planes plunge into the Twin Towers and, bizarrely for me, I had a mini epiphany about wanting to do something more meaningful with my life, and quit my job that day. I started working for the UK Coalition of People Living with HIV (UKC). It was glorious. I was surrounded by fabulous people living unashamedly with HIV.

Consuming information and sharing knowledge

I began writing for Positive Nation, the UKC publication by people with HIV for people with HIV. It was a tremendous glossy publication, edited by ludicrously clever veteran HIV activist Gus Cairns. I had a regular column 'Sex and the Suburbs' – I wrote about living a full and fabulous life with HIV, challenging the stereotypes of women with HIV as passive and voiceless victims.

One pervasive misconception about women with HIV was that we couldn't have children. I challenged this by posing naked on the 2004 cover of Positive Nation seven months pregnant with my third son (fathered by husband number three). Reclining on a sheepskin rug, I gazed triumphantly and unashamedly into the camera, under the headline 'Baby Love: Supremely Positive Pregnancies.' I wrote the feature article, celebrating that women with HIV with access to treatment would almost certainly have children born free of HIV, that it was our right to have children if we so chose. Too often at that time women with HIV were led to believe this wasn't possible, with many coerced into terminating their pregnancies.

A year after the magazine came out, a woman with HIV wrote to me to say her doctor had almost persuaded her to have an abortion, but she'd read my article and decided to keep her baby (who incidentally didn't have HIV, so middle finger up to that rubbish doctor). Although the majority of the feedback about my cover and feature was fabulous, I had received some vicious hate communication (even before internet trolling was a thing, so I guess I was before my time), accusing me of glamourising HIV, so reading that my article had made a difference and potentially saved a life somehow made it all worthwhile.

Intrusive side effects and drug resistance

Although there was effective treatment at that time, many people I worked with were affected by nasty side effects from their medication, such as gastro problems, lipodystrophy and peripheral neuropathy. Although I was fortunate not to have any of these, I was on a combination that had potential central nervous system side effects. I would wake up exhausted from vivid dreams, one a graphic sex dream about Saddam Hussein. Disturbing perhaps, but I recollect he was rather skilled for an evil dictator. I developed resistance to that drug and another in my combination during my pregnancy. Initially, I was told it happened because I wasn't taking my medication properly, something I would never do, particularly during my pregnancy when protecting my baby was my absolute priority. Later it was confirmed that it was likely due to my pregnancy size and that the hospital should have been monitoring the drug levels in my blood. Yet I had been blamed, as so often is the case for black women.

Black women with HIV often face intersecting forms of stigma, discrimination and disadvantage. I'm conscious my economic privilege and accent shields me from of some of the horrors experienced by some of my migrant sisters living with HIV in the UK, but I'm not entirely immune. I was diagnosed with an aggressive form of breast cancer in 2012, now with four children, and again faced with the devastating possibility of not living to see them grow up. I sat in the consultation room desperately trying to grasp the implications of triple negative breast cancer and a 5cm tumour, relayed to me by the white, portly ageing oncologist. He eyed me with a cloying mix of fascination and disgust, asking how I got HIV. What I was doing to stop my husband catching it from me. He then sent me out of a room for a blood test, with 'HIV high risk' scrawled on the form. I complained and changed hospitals, but it's often at times like this, when we are at our most vulnerable in healthcare settings, that black women with HIV face stigma and discrimination.

A platform to talk about inequalities and systemic racism

Professionally, a high that stands out for me was delivering the keynote address at IAS 2021, the world's most influential meeting on HIV research. Yes, I admit I got a buzz from topping former German Chancellor Angela Merkel on the programme, but it was having the opportunity to highlight issues of global HIV inequality to an audience of over 6,000 people that was more important. It gave me the platform to raise awareness of the shocking inequity both between countries and also within them in HIV treatment, care and support, and to discuss systemic racism at a time when the anti-woke agenda silences many of us, who are sometimes accused of having chips on our shoulders. Racism is real and blights the lives of so many of us, we shouldn't be afraid to call it out.

Another professional high is producing and hosting aidsmapLIVE, an award-winning broadcast discussion series for a global audience of people living with HIV. I've had incredible members of the HIV community, including the authors of this book, share their important insights, along with leading clinicians and policy-makers, including Winnie Byanyima, Executive Director of UNAIDS.

The professional highs pale into insignificance compared to the personal high since my HIV diagnosis of having two more extraordinary children, Ben and Tallulah, who make me proud every day, along with my other two sons Tom and James, and having the opportunity of living in an often chaotic but joyous multigenerational household that includes my mother Rita, my ultimate hero and inspiration.

During my HIV journey, the relationships with the most meaning to me include the sisterhood of other women living with HIV, whose friendship, support and empathy has been incredibly important. I'm fortunate that my family, including my children (my second son has become an influential HIV activist himself!), my mother and aunt, have been incredibly supportive throughout my HIV journey, as has my very best friend Julia, who I've known since before my diagnosis. It's taken a while to get here, but my relationship with myself, valuing who I am and what I've achieved, recognising that HIV is not a barrier to continuing to do better, is very important.

I'm conscious that coming from a Caribbean community, particularly being Black British, my experiences may differ from those of people from African communities living with HIV, but I think there is more that unifies us than divides us. I think we've learnt that we need to be meaningfully involved, we need to lead and design services and drive polices that are for us. Too often we've been wheeled out as case studies in media interviews, alongside white 'experts'. I think this needs to stop and instead we should have black people with HIV in the media as informed and empowered experts in our own rights, as so many of us are.

Although I've worked in the HIV sector for 20 years in various roles for various organisations, as an advocate, activist and public speaker, a few things stand out for me as key achievements. I'm proud of the impact I had as a writer at Positive Nation, challenging the stereotypes about women with HIV in my regular columns, as well as my notorious pregnancy feature, and hearing that at least one life was saved, by a mother with HIV defying the misguided advice to terminate her pregnancy against her wishes, after reading the column. I'm proud of the difference I've made in getting accurate yet engaging and empowering information about HIV to communities who are often ignored, through the broadcasts I've hosted and produced, particularly aidsmapLIVE, (with episodes being watched over 800,000 times!), and the video content I've produced, featuring people with HIV not as case studies, but sharing their important insights. If I had to try to squeeze my achievements in together as a soundbite I guess I could say it's the role I've played in fighting the health inequities experienced by women and people of colour with HIV – something for which I've recently been invited to become a Fellow of the Royal Society of Arts. I hope I will continue to make a difference.

We need to lead and drive services and policies that are for us.

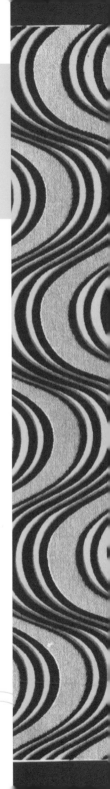

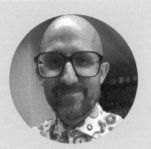

COMMON THREADS: A PROFESSIONAL AND PERSONAL JOURNEY

Tristan Barber

remember the first AIDS cases from the USA and the UK being presented by one of my schoolteachers, probably in the early 1980s. This was at a time when I was internally starting to acknowledge my own sexuality; that I wasn't quite the same as people around me and at a time when being gay wasn't such a visible thing. Through secondary school, I don't remember hearing so much about HIV. I grew up in Cornwall, quite remote from London and the main focus of the epidemic, so I don't remember it being talked about that much. I do remember a documentary called Common Threads about the AIDS quilt that was narrated by Dustin Hoffman, and I watched over and over and over again. I remember watching the 'In Bed with Madonna' documentary, where she did a tribute to Keith Haring who had died of AIDS. Things started to feel like they were a little bit closer to me, particularly because I was naming my sexuality more.

I remember taking Common Threads to show my Sixth Form because they hadn't heard of it or seen it. People became very upset by some of the stories that were told. What that documentary did very well was knitting together stories of different people from different backgrounds, including people who had acquired HIV through blood products, young haemophiliacs. It was very powerful for those who, at that time, thought it was very much a gay disease.

The night before my medical school interview, I travelled to London to stay with my aunt and uncle. That was the day that Freddie Mercury died. I got into medical school and I remember moving to London, and trying to grow as a gay man. This was a time when people were still in a state of shock about the HIV epidemic. We didn't have triple combination therapy. It was difficult to get to know your elders, because they were so directly affected by AIDS. For those of us that moved to London in the 1990s were a generation that had not been directly affected. As a result, it took a bit of time to get grounded and find people in the city.

A space to think

In 1996, during my summer holidays from medical school, I ended up working as a secretary for six weeks at the Royal Free Hospital for Professor Margaret Johnson, working in HIV and writing letters about people who were on dual nucleoside therapy. All the doctors were just back from the World AIDS Conference in Vancouver, and they were very excited about triple therapy. It was at this point that I started thinking that I might have found a career in medicine that would suit me.

I also spent some time in Kenya in 1999 with a friend who runs an NGO there. I worked in HIV centres in Western Kenya and in the Rift Valley. When I came back to London, I was thinking, I'm not sure I want to go to Africa just yet. I'm not sure I want to do more medical exams. I need to do a bit more growing up. In that growing up phase, I let my career lapse for a year or two, as I needed some space to grow personally, and I thought I wanted to do things in medicine that were more acute, maybe anaesthetics, or accident emergency medicine. It was looking like becoming a six-month career gap when, at the last minute, I found a job in sexual health.

It was 2002 and I enjoyed that job so much. I had such a good time, in fact, at the departmental summer party I went home with another member of staff, and we had unprotected sex that led to my sero-conversion. The irony is not lost on me that I acquired HIV during my first junior job in sexual health!

This was though, a pivotal moment for me as I became convinced that was what I wanted to do as a career. A personal and professional journey started there. I also knew I had to gain the medical exams that I had been avoiding, so I started my route back into working in HIV.

Finding a way to separate the personal and professional

I had been avoiding working in the HIV sector, perhaps due to my own narrow viewpoint about the epidemic affecting mainly white gay men at certain HIV centres. I wasn't sure I wanted my working life and my personal life to be so close.

I was lucky that there was much more diversity in the first job I got in London. I was on the ward looking after sick Africans and gay men, but a lot of sick Africans diagnosed with AIDS. Being back in that environment motivated me to get back into HIV.

When I started in 2002, the treatment environment was fairly exciting. We'd had triple therapy since 1996, although the treatments were fairly toxic and we were managing a legacy of antiretroviral toxicity, AIDS-defining problems, but also people who had acquired resistance. I think this was a perfect time to learn about antiretroviral resistance in a way that I don't think junior doctors learn about so well now.

When I got my first proper HIV job, it was a research post. Everyone thinks that after 1996 things were rosy, but between 2000 and 2007 we ran out of drugs again. There was a real stall. White people had acquired resistance during sequential monotherapy. People were being treated with low genetic barrier regimens in the late 1990s, thinking it was wonderful. Then they acquired toxicity and liver injuries, and then suddenly they acquired more resistance as treatment failed. As doctors we were stuck with Kaletra (which we know to have nasty gastric side effects), some old nucleosides and T20 (an injection twice a day). When I started the research job, we were running the Optima Study, which was just basically throwing in five, six, seven drugs, any drugs to see if you could get people re-suppressed, and if doing this was better.

Conservatism, controversy and HIV medication

Sexual health and HIV is a good specialty for pushing boundaries and inclusivity, but medicine can still be quite conservative at times. HIV care is fantastic, due to the involvement of people living with HIV helping to smash down so many barriers. I'm still shocked when I come across or work with more traditional colleagues, particularly with issues around boundaries for younger LGBTQ+ colleagues coming into the specialty. The barriers are down when you first work in a sexual health clinic – very different from working in cardiology or surgery – because people are talking about sex, they're talking about drugs, they're talking about things that are not talked about in a lot of medicine. As result, people often find a niche. They're in their 20s, the barriers, the boundaries are fluid, and sometimes it takes time to rebalance your professional life, and ensure clear delineation from your personal one.

There was a time when rather than supporting people who were having those boundary issues, some people were 'removed'. They were sidelined from a specialty, they weren't promoted, they weren't encouraged to apply for jobs, they weren't kept in training, it was just deemed that they were not appropriate. It coincided with the emergence of new sexual networking apps for phones. This was the first time I really saw that although you think you're in a permissive environment, there can be some persistent old conservative attitudes – that really shocked me. These people actually needed support and help from the people whose job it was to look after people who were reporting drug use and sex. We were supporting them, but we couldn't support our own colleagues who were going through similar challenges. I found that really difficult.

Being part of a global community

As your HIV career develops you realise it's the global community that you are interacting with. The fact that we really deliver person-centred care in a way that challenges so much of the rest of medicine. We've been trying at the moment within HIV care to use person-centred language for submitted abstracts and research papers. This still leads to occasional conflict from people who think we should still use terms like 'patients' rather than 'people with HIV', for example.

A highlight of working as a team is working alongside people who experience the condition that we are treating and supporting. That really helps you get through the tough things, keeping people at the centre of what we're doing.

HIV conferences all around the world are exciting. I have spoken at conferences in Durban, Mexico City and the USA, as well as others closer to home. We get to go to these fantastic amazing conferences, see incredible people, experience incredible local culture.

For me, the real gift of my job is definitely sitting with someone who's newly diagnosed and being able to tell them things that they think are magic are actually real; being able to tell them that they can have a normal life expectancy, they can have children and they can suppress their virus and not transmitted the virus sexually. The fact that the science allows us to deliver such truly life-changing information to people, that's a real privilege and a real one-to-one connection.

Global attention: a community not seen

African people affected by HIV were not talked about at the beginning of the epidemic. It wasn't the Black Africans that hit the headlines, it was the white, cis-gendered gay men in affluent North America, in Los Angeles and New York. African communities have always been on the backfoot. I remember coming to this conclusion at a World AIDS Day event.

I remembered those awful discussions in the early days; why do so many people in sub-Saharan Africa have HIV? Why is the prevalence so high? Why is it spread heterosexually? It's not the same as in Europe and North America. It must be their sexual networks. It must be the way that they have relationships and multiple marriages. No, it's just the fact that it's been spreading in Africa for 80 years, probably before you noticed the white tip of the iceberg poking its head out in North America. In Africa the spread had gone unchecked for so long, because average life expectancy was lower and so deaths in young adults were less noticeable.

That story is not, I think, still well known. There was less media attention; they just don't treat human beings with equal worth. What has been powerful is that since the first AIDS cases came to the public attention, the power has been in bringing people together. It wasn't easy in the beginning. People didn't necessarily know what would work. There was always this assumption that Black Africans would be religious and therefore judgemental about people's sexuality. Actually, among the things that HIV has delivered for us is not only more public discussion of sexuality, but also broader issues of migration, race, and equity of healthcare access as a human right. HIV highlighted the huge impact on public health of not treating people equally, a lesson we are still not learning now, even with the Covid-19 pandemic.

Some of my sadness in recent years is that the togetherness has been slightly lost. I see that in the prevention discussions. Pre-exposure prophylaxis (PrEP) is clearly successful. The rollout in the UK has heavily focused on men who have sex with men, and who have seen rapidly decreasing rates of HIV transmission. This is to be celebrated, but we continue to see higher rates of transmission in heterosexuals, who are not white, even in metropolitan areas, just outside of central London, for example, people presenting with AIDS-defining conditions. We've lost that coalition of groups working together to ensure that everyone's awareness is raised at the same time. This is the sadness of recent years and needs to be corrected. I think in terms of fighting from an African perspective, it's women who have driven this. African male voices are starting too and need to be heard more and more. The advocacy work around vertical transmission has been great and the now the current advocacy work around breastfeeding. I think globally, what we're finding is how fantastic the fight back is. I think what Africans have done with HIV, in particular, is to push the conservatism of medicine. They pushed on those doors that needed to be broken down, that were not areas of attention for the white men running the research studies at the time. This is a story that's replicated in many areas of the world, many areas of medicine, but has been so tremendously important, particularly given that HIV worldwide is a disease that predominantly affects women and predominantly affects Africans.

A community of grown-ups

I did my growing up as a gay man after my HIV diagnosis, and the particular relationships that strengthened that were a group of friends I found at the Royal Vauxhall Tavern, which is a pub in South London. I found a community of grownups who also knew how to have fun, many of whom were living with HIV, with whom you could have honest, adult discussions around sex and just growing up gay. My career definitely became more successful because for having that community.

Over time, the boundaries of work and play would be crossed. People would phone me at weekends and at all hours of the night asking about HIV risk, treatments, post-exposure prophylaxis, or what could they do about friends who were overdoing drugs. It became difficult to get rest and, for me, to not be a doctor at the weekends in addition to all week.

As my career developed, I spent less time at the Tavern, but I remain extremely grateful for the family that supported, encouraged and, indeed, loved me there. There was no time off for me, but that dense family feeling across those 10 years really changed me from being a sort of mid-20s child into a much more functioning professional and happier adult.

One of the things that could have been done differently is that the research community should have got behind the inclusion of women in trials at a much earlier stage. Only now do we have powerful advocates talking about and calling for the meaningful involvement of women in research. If you look at the UK, we have some really strong female HIV consultants, many of whom started their careers at a time when most consultants were men. Women really had to fight to break down some of those barriers and now they are in the driving seat and can push for inclusion, something that could have been done a lot sooner.

Not everything will happen in a timeline or in a way that you want it to.

TODAY I ...

Today I say goodbye to feeling guilty
when I take a day off work.
Goodbye to self-doubt, negative energy and
chaos in my life.
Goodbye to procrastination, to dillydallying
and putting things off.
I say goodbye to saying sorry,
Old habits that cause self-harm.
Replacing with better behaviour,
which I practise more frequently
Today I say hello,
to sorting stuff out,
actioning stuff and my new list
of things to do.
Hello to a potential new lover, hello to my free life.
Hello world. What else do you have to offer me?
I say helloooo to new beginnings!
Hello sunshine, hello living freely,
Hello life, I fully embrace you!

Group poem

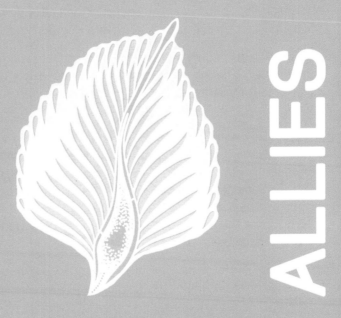

ALLIES

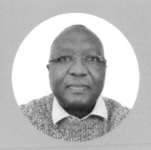

ENGINEERING HIV PREVENTION: THE GRASSROOTS APPROACH

Badru Male

I am a Ugandan living in the UK since 1990. I left Uganda at the age of 19 after my A-levels and came to Europe to study engineering. I got a scholarship, but due to political instability I remained abroad, waiting for calmness in my home country. One thing led to another and I never actually returned. I graduated in 1981 as a civil engineer and worked in North Africa and in the UK for a total of 10 years.

In early 1990s, there was an outbreak of advanced HIV cases in the Ugandan community living in the UK and this needed an immediate response. It was of a great concern to all of the Ugandan community and education and raising awareness about HIV prevention and support for people already living with HIV was much needed.

I registered with a newly founded voluntary organisation, the Uganda AIDS Action Fund as a member of the board of trustees and responsible for volunteers' recruitment and management. Most of the activities were geared towards raising awareness, information dissemination and advocacy.

In 1994, I was invited to Croydon in South London by a group of Ugandans who had another idea in mind. This was not about primary prevention, but support for those already living with HIV. At this time, there was a lot of stigma around living with HIV such that people affected lived in self-isolation, and in most cases their health deteriorated so much that they need practical as well as emotional support. This organisation was later known as the African Community Involvement Association and I was elected the first chairman of the board of trustees.

As I got more and more involved in the field of HIV prevention and support, I needed more knowledge on the condition itself and therefore I started to seek more information. I did a short counselling course at St Charles Hospital in West London that equipped me with basic knowledge about bereavement support and pre- and post-HIV test counselling and support.

In 1996, I spent most of the time in HIV prevention and support. Some of the earlier services developed were HIV support groups held in people's houses and one-to-one emotional support. I slowly moved from engineering to healthcare, and few years later I decided to get a qualification in the field. I registered for a two-year Health Studies course at St George's Medical School. This course equipped me with the knowledge and skills to deal with sociological issues of community health, health promotion, developing evidence-based projects, understanding health beliefs and population health. Another HIV-related course at Thames Valley University improved my knowledge of HIV, immunology, pharmacology and HIV specific health promotion.

The devastation of a diagnosis

In the African communities, where my activities were concentrated in the early 1990s, there was a very high mortality rate due to late diagnosis. The first main aim of the services I developed were focused on reducing the mortality rate, which meant encouraging early diagnosis. Then in the mid-1990s, an effective combination therapy treatment reduced the number of people dying from HIV-related illnesses.

The next task was to encourage people to adhere to these treatments. People had started developing drug resistance associated with non-adherence. Actually at that time we called it treatment compliancy. An issue then was tolerance to medication. There were so many pills to take and due to the high toxicity of the medication, there were severe side effects that put people off taking the medication religiously. Some of these adverse effects included peripheral neuropathy, lipodystrophy, early onset of conditions such as diabetes, rheumatoid arthritis and gastric problems. Then, later as people lived longer with HIV, they experienced early onset of old age symptoms such as dementia and weaknesses in body organs and senses.

The evolving needs of the community

In the early years of HIV in communities there were many people dying. This was one of my lows. In many cases, we were just looking on to see people passing away with nothing that could be done. We used to attend three of four funerals a week. I saw many people suffering and HIV-related stigma was so high.

The changing priorities in commissioning processes also frustrated many emerging services, especially as HIV-related conditions started to be felt in new communities. HIV education and knowledge have been very dynamic in that, as progress in managing the condition improved, services that mattered had to change to be in line with the changing needs of the community.

However, as drugs for combination therapy became available and more were licensed, the situation changed and that was the first hope and high excitement of being able to keep people alive. The start of HIV advocacy and encouragement to have treatment-expert patients, to support people who were newly diagnosed was also a new high. HIV treatment advocacy became a top activity, giving people living with HIV a voice and participation in decisions affecting their health. This important step has changed the way HIV management is conducted and I pay tribute to the pioneers of HIV treatment advocacy at HIV i-Base, National Aids Trust, NAM and the UK-CAB.

The importance of and relationship advice for the future generations

I have been impressed by the relationship of healthcare professionals with the patients over the years. Doctors, consultants and specialist nurses have been key in the management of HIV both in hospitals and the extended services in the community. The voluntary sector has been and still is key in engaging with communities in both prevention and support for people living with HIV. Now that we talk about combination prevention, the triangle of healthcare professionals, the voluntary sector and the service users have to work together to create a synergy of services to achieve the 2030 targets of eliminating the transmission of HIV.

HIV has no boundaries and therefore services have to include everyone. In the beginning, only targeted prevention worked and some communities were left out. These are the communities that are highly affected years later. Services have to be developed with a view to eliminate inequalities and maintain involvement for all. Inequalities are also seen in the commissioning and in the delivery processes. Most important now, we need to move further from addressing inequalities to looking at addressing inequity. The number of new diagnoses is falling in one group of society but increasing in the other.

Which one of this group needs more intervention or more funding? This is where the inequity concept comes from, so this is one way of doing things differently.

When I was young, there was nothing called sex and relationship education. All we learnt was reproduction that was being taught with a giggle here and there. Sex and relationship education was a subject for the adults. In people's home, sex was never discussed. It was taboo. No wonder some people started having sex at a young age without knowing about pregnancy and sexually transmitted infections. In my primary school, I remember girls got pregnant at 14, 15 or 16 depending on when they started school or how many classes they repeated. Boys used to have sex for fun. The bigger the number of sexual partners, the more proud you were.

We have to promote sex and relationship education in schools starting from a young age. In that way, children will grow up with responsibility for their sexual lives. I have involved my younger children in sex and relationship education. They discuss with me anything about their sex life openly and this should be the same with all parents. We have to normalise sex education in order to tackle stigma associated with sex and sexually transmitted infections and conditions, and promote support and care for those living with the conditions.

HIV testing in all community settings

In the 30 years of working in the sector, I have contributed to the reduction of HIV-related mortality and morbidity. I have encouraged many people, especially from the ethnic minority backgrounds, to get involved in the HIV sector and make an impact on educating the communities, support and care and continue to encourage other to get involved. I have contributed to having stronger and effective advocacy teams and individuals. The UK-CAB had a few of us Black African advocates in the 1990s and now there are many and they are the administrators. I have trained over 100 HIV treatment advocates in and around the UK. I have trained HIV treatment advocates in other European cities, including Amsterdam and Brussels. This is something that I am extremely proud of. I have encouraged people from other minority ethnic backgrounds to get involved and recently developed a resource specifically for the Muslim communities, the publication HIV Knowledge and Islam (published by Positive East) in order to involve Muslim clergy in the fight to achieve the 2030 UN targets. My aim is to focus on reducing the number of undiagnosed HIV by working with all communities to encourage HIV testing in all community settings.

I am very grateful to the colleagues, brothers and sisters that I have worked with in the past 30 years of working in the HIV sector. I am very proud to be part of the relationship fostered with all professionals, service users and volunteers in the sector. I have learnt a lot from other providers and I have learnt a lot about different communities. The skills I have gained over time are life skills and I am privileged to have been in a position to pass them on to other people. I do not regret changing my career from engineering to public health.

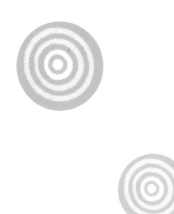

HIV prevention begins with an individual. Let's all get involved.

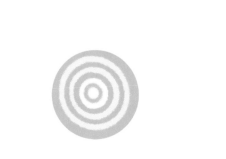

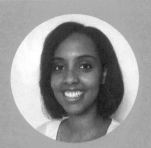

WOULD YOU LIKE TO BE A DOCTOR? I CAN HELP PEOPLE STAY WELL IN DIFFERENT WAYS

Chamut Kifetew

I was born and raised in Kenya, East Africa, to two wonderful Ethiopian parents. I always had a keen interest in helping people stay healthy and well, especially women and girls, but when my parents asked me, at age six, if I wanted to be a doctor, I looked at them horrified and said, 'I don't want to look at blood all day!' The TV medical drama, ER, was a household favourite at the time. I reasoned that I would have to help people stay healthy in a different way, and became very interested in public health.

I moved to Melbourne, Australia, in 2010 to pursue academic studies in public health, and soon after joined the local Women's Service to raise awareness among women and girls from key communities about potentially harmful cultural practices such as female genital cutting. I moved to Birmingham, UK, to develop my career in public health and ended up specialising in community health promotion with an HIV and sexual health focus.

I feel really passionately about health issues that are seen as taboo by many societies. Often they are fully preventable and treatable, but many people suffer to the point of serious illness due to ignorance born from the shame and stigma of speaking up about it. I want to be one of the people who raises awareness of these issues and helps dispel this ignorance, so as many people as possible know the facts and can protect their health and live happy, well and fulfilled lives. The HIV sector does this at its core and has had so much of an impact on people affected by the condition that I have been proud to be part of it.

Watching HIV care evolve

When I first got involved in the HIV landscape in 2016, PrEP was not available to people, research was just emerging on the benefits of early initiation of treatment, the general public didn't know about the 'Can't Pass It On' or U=U message, and funding for HIV organisations' support services was being cut left, right and centre. There was so much potential, but unfortunately so many challenges at the same time.

My work has focused largely on HIV prevention over the last seven years. In that time, it has been a key highlight to have PrEP become routinely available on the NHS.

However, at the same time, as a woman of African heritage, it has been incredibly demoralising to see how gender and ethnic inequities in access to PrEP (and broader HIV services, such as testing) persist and in fact are baked into the system. It seems that women and people of Black African ethnicity are always an afterthought, and policies and services are not designed with these groups in mind. They are invisible right until the end – at which point, there is a scramble and a few resources thrown around to try and catch up, and it rarely works, because the system was never designed for these groups in the first place.

This is despite women, and particularly Black African women, having among the highest rates of HIV diagnoses year on year compared to any other group.

Witnessing the powerful U=U message become a global message of hope, as well as a framework to address structural inequities and advocate for treatment access as a basic right and more, has been a career high. I hope that this movement continues and builds so that globally every person living with HIV has full access to HIV treatment and health professionals and members of the public alike know about the message and HIV stigma becomes a thing of the past once and for all.

The fabric of HIV care

Working in the HIV sector is unique and wonderful because of the dynamic, passionate and caring individuals who make up its fabric – clinicians, commissioners, community advocates, service users, health promotion workers and more. Nearly everyone I've had the pleasure of working with has been united by a common goal of ending new transmissions and helping everyone living with HIV to be well.

As a person working in the sector, there have been certain lessons that I've learnt along the way. It's important to keep on top of key evidence as it comes out, because HIV medicine and how it affects people changes rapidly. What was true five or even two years ago may not be true now or two years from now. Keeping an eye on the evidence allows a person in the sector to be effective and realistic and achieve maximum impact. It also helps the person advocate on issues that are relevant and helps to futureproof a person's work.

Collaboration and coproduction are key processes that everyone should embed as their way of working. It helps ensure that initiatives are relevant and will get the buy-in they need to succeed. Regular communication with stakeholders is key to getting them on board, and it is a two-way street. It is important to seek understanding of how you can help meet the goals of your stakeholders, not just your own aims. Where those goals align is where plans will succeed.

Finally, as a project manager, it would be remiss of me to not mention the value of planning. It seems an obvious thing, but some may be surprised how easy it is to jump into running an initiative or service without properly planning each aspect and monitoring progress throughout the process. For me, planning is essential to success.

I am proud of having led and supported a sector development programme over many years to build the capacity of the HIV sector to be more aware of the latest research and key issues, including equity of access. I have always been a staunch advocate for women and people of Black African ethnicity and addressing the gaps in prevention and treatment services they experience. One example that I am especially proud of is advocating for better PrEP access for these groups through a 2020 PrEP campaign programme I was involved in called PrEP Protects. I presented the results of this campaign at the Spring 2021 BHIVA/BASHH conference and was awarded the Martin Fisher Award for best community oral abstract presentation.

We are all different pieces of the puzzle, and no one piece can make the big picture.

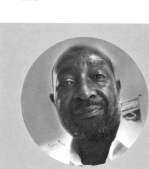

AN AFTERTHOUGHT FROM ZIMBABWE TO LONDON: FALLING INTO HIV CARE

Charles Mazhude

When I was in Zimbabwe, I worked in various areas, including the management of sexually transmitted infections (STIs). Before I moved to the UK, I remember being struck by the volume of STIs that we had in the city. Around the time HIV started rearing its head, I remember wondering what the impact of HIV might be on my country. In my final medical school exam, I wrote the answer HIV in one of the questions as an afterthought, because we were beginning to see HIV in the care setting.

As a young registrar joining the sector in 1996, we had dedicated hospital wards for patients with HIV and those with AIDS. From a medical point of view, we were doing incredible medicine. There was so much desperation. There were lots of experimental therapies going on. It was a very frenetic time on the wards. You would find men with lungs clogged up with Kaposi's sarcoma and all the usual infections. Then before my eyes, over one or two years, I saw the wards start to empty. I remember a colleague coming back from Vancouver, talking about protease inhibitors, which totally revolutionised what was going on. At the time we were battling to understand how we were going to deal with tolerability, which was a major issue. We almost had to sacrifice that for efficacy in terms of whether the treatments worked or not. We all began to learn the craft of antiretroviral therapy.

You will hear stories of people having to suck ice cubes and drink all sorts of things to make the medications palatable. People were also exploring ways to manage the diarrhoea, which was relentless.

Over the years, antiretroviral therapy evolved. We had a few more drugs available, so we could start paying more and more attention to tolerability. It improved and then the battle against resistance started. Eventually, we got to the point where we could manage most patients who had resistance. Now, we've arrived at the stage where tolerability and efficacy are taken for granted. It's really about how we look at the long-term benefits to the individual, as well as how convenient this is for the people who are on treatment, and hopefully, at some point, a cure.

Finding a supportive mentor: are you happy to see an African doctor?

I was a young black doctor in the HIV field in South London Hospital where there was a large ethnic mix of people. The key relationship for me that actually led to me getting a post in this large south London centre, where I was able to do my training, was with Anton Pozniak, a leading HIV doctor. His encouragement was key. There were very few other clinicians that I knew who were African and working in HIV. I had lots of relationships with other organisations that were working within the HIV sector. Because I represented a slightly different demographic – a lot of my colleagues in the field were men who have sex with men (MSM) – I was looking at the African community. I could see how the HIV epidemic was evolving on the African continent in terms of the types of patients we had seen over the years. We started seeing people from East and Central Africa, a total deluge of Zimbabweans at one point and then that moved away, then we had a few other Southern African countries. Over time, we eventually ended up with more patients coming from West Africa. I could see this happening, immigration patterns emerging and being important. There was this evolution that I could see in terms of how the HIV epidemic was affecting the African continent and also the attitudes of newly diagnosed people who were from those communities, according to how the HIV pandemic had affected their particular countries. In terms of key relationships, it was obviously the clinicians that impacted on me, but also the patients that I interacted with. I felt that to some extent I was perhaps able to offer something slightly different than for the other conditions I provided care for.

Some people might not have wanted to see an African doctor, but stigma was an issue. In fact, interestingly, when I got appointed to start a new service in Lewisham, I was told, 'There's going to be lots of African patients. Are they going to be happy to see an African doctor?' It concerned me a bit, in terms of how is this going to work? But, actually, 20 years on it's been quite the opposite. I think cultural appropriateness has been quite important for some of our clients. It's not everyone's cup of tea, but it's actually very useful with the patients that I've been managing over the years.

Doctor knows best: developing advocacy

You treat people who are coming from a background where people do not advocate for themselves. Traditionally, there is a 'doctor knows best' kind of approach in our African practice, so it was really useful to have certain key people say, 'Look, we've got to make a stand for the African cause.' HIV medicine in general, has been one of those areas where patient-led advocacy has made a huge impact in terms of how HIV management has evolved, and has led medicine in general, in terms of acknowledgment and realising how useful it can be to have patients involved at every stage. It's really worked in the gay community, who were very strong in terms of fighting for their rights. The African community wasn't nearly as vocal. I think we learnt a lot from that advocacy within our own communities. We decided to confront stigma.

Peer support networks were critical. They helped the sanity of a lot of people dealing with not only HIV but also feelings of being 'other' in this country and away from home. You're an immigrant, you're trying to get a job, you're trying to get your papers sorted, managing uncertainty … and then you've got this very stigmatising condition. The formation of multiple support organisations was vital. In terms of supporting people, as a clinician it is useful to know that there are issues beyond antiretrovirals, viral loads and CD4. People need social support and it is vital to be able to signpost people to this.

Finding a 360-degree view of the world

It starts at the level of the individual. People living with HIV need to get to a point where as an individual they are taking responsibility for their health and advocating for it; so when they see their clinician, they can acknowledge that there are things that need to be discussed. We are now at the stage where people with HIV are getting older and are beginning to get arthritis and diabetes, and everybody's getting high blood pressure. We need to make sure people can self-manage and have control over their health. They need a 360-degree view of what's going on so that they can prioritise their health in their own way.

We need more education and self-empowerment, with advocacy organisations working in a more joined-up fashion so that we can continue to utilise the available resources – working together, self-education and awareness are all important. Coordinated work is important, because I think that even since the days of AHPN, there has been a lot of politics, which is not helpful in terms of finding common ground and priorities in HIV care.

Being an African doctor has been an important contribution to the sector and at a critical time when there weren't many of us to start with, in terms of diversity of clinicians in HIV care. At every meeting that needed a black clinician, I was able to speak and provide a diverse opinion.

I think the advent of antiretroviral therapy was mind-blowing. It was quite something in the whole scheme of things and everything since has been a refinement of that point; where we should focus, developing a single pill, and now we might be doing an injection or two.

The other thing that is remarkable about my experience has been the learning that comes from the patient's point of view – this has had a relevant part to play in terms of directing the role I have and is something other areas of care could learn from.

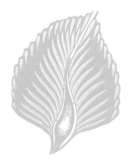 People living with HIV are the experts when it comes to the care they need.

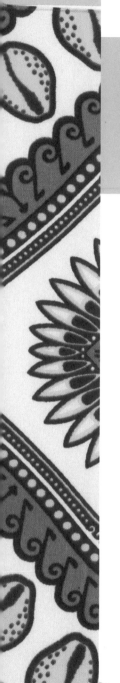

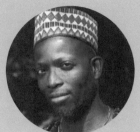

SUICIDE, STIGMA AND A PASSION TO FIGHT HIV-RELATED STIGMA

Cheikh Traore

In the year 1998, soon after completing a postgraduate degree, the HIV sector offered me my first volunteering opportunity in London. I joined the Food Chain as kitchen assistant in its Hackney kitchen in East London. Our job was to prepare nutritious meals that would be delivered to people living with HIV in the Greater London area. I was unemployed and this experience gave me a sense of purpose, free lunches and a useful way to spend my weekends. A year later, I saw an announcement for volunteers in another HIV charity; Body Positive had opened its drop-in centre in Soho and needed volunteers to manage a new modern learning centre. I volunteered for two years with these two HIV organisations and since then I have not left the HIV sector.

There are multiple reasons why I was drawn to work in the HIV sector; and 20 years on my passion has not faltered. When AIDS was first described, I had just joined medical school in Dakar, Senegal. I had a patient diagnosed with AIDS in 1987 and I still remember the panic in the ward that followed among students and medical personnel. The patient later committed suicide. The experience marked my conscience and ignited my passion to understand and fight HIV-related stigma.

I grew up in a family of political activists, where both Mom and Dad made huge personal sacrifices to fight for social justice and democracy in Africa. That is where I inherited a passion for pan-Africanist ideals and women's liberation. Coming to terms with my own homosexuality in my mid-20s during medical school happened after years of questioning about sex and intellectual curiosity for all things related to sexuality. In the late 1980s and early 1990s, during my university years, HIV was not associated with homosexuality in West Africa. Only once I saw a short video jingle with a message about HIV and homosexuality, and that was in Côte d'Ivoire. However, thanks to my own personal reading, I knew that HIV had caused a lot of devastation in communities of gay and bisexual men in Europe and North America. After medical school, I knew that my interest was to work in public health and particularly in policy. I currently work freelance as a policy adviser in various countries. Policy work is where my passion for social justice, politics, pan-Africanism and gay liberation all come nicely together.

The myriad community groups: volunteering in the HIV sector and then finding work

After years of volunteering in the London HIV sector, I got my first job offer in 1999 at Terrence Higgins Trust as a Health Promotion Officer for African men. At the time, there were huge imbalances in terms of access to HIV care. I was working mostly with African communities and service users tended to be diagnosed in the late stages of disease compared to their British/white counterparts. Gender inequalities within African communities were stark; many HIV services hardly saw African men, which is why my position was created. HIV service providers in London would see a lot more women diagnosed often through antenatal care, but they had major challenges in reaching African men, who either did not trust service providers because of fears around immigration status or who refused to attend services and be confronted with gay men or transgender people in the same reception areas. Homophobia was rife, so services that were designed around the needs of gay men had a hard time reaching African men. Working with African men was a tale of challenging social marginalisation caused by racism, the legal limbos of asylum status, low self-esteem and a lot of despair. These factors took prominence over and above the virus itself, despite medical advances and the arrival of effective combination therapy.

The highs of my work were the experiences of working with a myriad of community groups, originating from various parts of the continent. Almost every weekend my team had invitations from community groups who wanted to discuss HIV; mostly Somalis, Ugandans, Rwandans, Congolese, Zimbabweans and some West Africans. As a pan-Africanist, London was heaven – a fascinating microcosm of so many diverse communities with different belief systems who were now redefined as Black African by virtue of living in the UK. Discussing HIV with African communities inevitably brought up the issues of race, immigration and asylum, so we had to be very careful in the way we used communication channels to reach communities. Debates about race equality in the healthcare system were beginning to gain prominence in the late 1990s, and this has been of great help in my work to raise awareness of cultural competence among healthcare providers.

Condom use, conspiracy theorists and HIV denial

There were lots of memorable downsides. I remember being invited to discuss HIV with a group young Somalis, on the condition that I did not to discuss condom use. Another time, I was invited to speak at a huge community event within the compounds of a major London teaching hospital. As the event started, I realised it was funded and organised by treatment denialists and conspiracy theorists, lecturing about the virus that was designed to wipe out the Black race. Such events were very common in the late 1990s and I later met a few treatment denialists even within the HIV sector. I also remember instances of rejection; a known Black radio station refused to air our World AIDS Day interview because African accents were 'not cool'!

At the Terrence Higgins Trust, there was a team of gay men managing a vibrant national partnership called CHAPS (Community HIV/AIDS Prevention Strategy). We became friends and I also got to familiarise myself with health promotion efforts for gay and bisexual men in England and Wales. Until 2001, there was literally zero debate about the needs of African gay and bisexual men within the HIV sector. I was facing a dilemma. I had a vibrant social life with fellow gay and bisexual Africans, but their experiences were absent from all our community work. I was also attending a few services designed for black gay men organised by GMFA, London Lighthouse and PACE (Project for Advocacy, Counseling and Education). They had innovative approaches where mental health wellbeing was firmly embedded in health promotion work. That is where I met Dennis Carney, a mental health coach who made a huge impact on my personal journey to self-acceptance. After much reflection, I took the decision to come out as a gay man during the annual African men's health seminar organised by Camden NHS Trust. It was a memorable event, and I am glad that many more African men were able to follow suit and be open about their sexuality within those community events. Thanks to Simon Nelson of the CHAPS team and Rhon Reynolds from the African HIV Policy Network (AHPN), we designed a plan to create more visibility for Black gay men in the HIV sector.

All along my journey in the UK HIV sector, there were many individuals who boosted my motivation and helped me to develop myself to learn more and take on even more professional responsibilities. I owe a lot to the activists. There were two types: the vocal angry activists and the quiet ones. At Body Positive (1998–99) I was a volunteer under the supervision of Jo Pease and Robert Fieldhouse (quiet activists). I still owe them a lot and admire their selflessness and dedication to the cause. At the Terrence Higgins Trust, I was lucky to work under giants in the fight against HIV, starting with Lisa Power. She was not the angry activist type, and not quiet either. Her enormous sense of humour made it a joy to work alongside her. She willingly gave long history lessons about the struggles of the queer movement, as well as the HIV movement. I met great leaders within the NHS, like Dorothy Mukasa who were greatly committed to the fight against HIV within African communities and who founded the AHPN. AHPN was able to attract rare gems in both policy and community work. I forever remain grateful to the trailblazers like Winnie Sseruma and Henry Mumbi who paved the way for the emancipation of people living with HIV, and constantly encouraged me to serve our communities.

Responding to the HIV crisis

The UK's HIV response in the years between 2000 and 2021 has not been sufficiently celebrated around the world. The UK is one of the few countries where the response took onboard the many intersecting dimensions of discrimination that communities affected by HIV experience. This experiment was done at great political risk, but it has borne many fruits. For many years, there was also a great deal of collaboration between HIV scientists, communities and the NHS. However, as medical treatment became more effective, the emphasis on community mobilisation seems to have dwindled. It will be a hard sell to rekindle the spirit of those years to face new pandemics such as monkeypox and Covid-19.

Currently I am working from my base in Lagos, Nigeria. I travel across the African continent mostly as a consultant on HIV, gender and human rights. What we did successfully in the UK 15 years ago in terms of addressing human rights intersections has only been recently adopted within global HIV policy. There is no doubt that my early experiences in the UK continue to have a huge influence on my professional approaches.

Being successful in the HIV sector requires a great deal of generosity and dedication, but above all it requires strong leadership skills in order to navigate a relatively small but complex sector. AHPN continues to be a major achievement for the community response to HIV in the UK. Unfortunately, I feel that a number of factors largely linked to leadership deficit and poor strategy have caused the AHPN gradually to lose relevance. I was a board member of the AHPN between 2006 and 2008 and I felt that with sufficient leadership skills I could have done a lot more to solve its internal crises.

We must raise awareness about the importance of cultural sensitivity and the need to embed anti-racist work within HIV and health promotion.

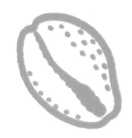

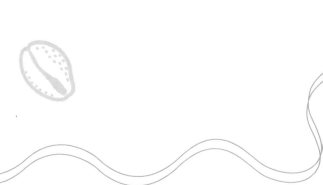

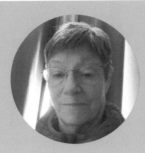

ALL ABOARD: THE ANGER AND PASSION IN HIV ACTIVISM

Elisabeth Crafer

Living in a rural area in the 1980s, I saw women had a raw deal regarding health services. Health professionals seemed to have little interest in women's health needs beyond prescribing a handful of tranquillisers, so I bought a 7-ton lorry from a car auction and converted it into a health information mobile for women that parked up in town centres, villages and workplaces. In the mobile, women shared experiences and created information based on their own experiences and questions. They changed services by demanding to be listened to.

My excitement in getting mainstream health services to respond to the voice and engagement of those long ignored, took me down the road of Manager of Hertsaid. This support service was formed by two gay men, bravely open about their status and mad as hell at the lack of services in a rural area. Here was a chance for integrating lived experience into services, for developing peer support. A chance to take the anger and passion needed for the beginning of a service into survivability without loss of direction. In 1998, after the organisation was successfully set up, I moved on to Positively Women/Positively UK and new adventures.

In truth, I lay some of the blame for my working in the world of HIV on Jon Grimshaw (an openly positive activist) who in 1988 spoke at the Lister Hospital in Stevenage about the engagement of people with HIV in research and care. It reminded me that as a woman who had bought and driven a lorry and as a parent who had survived the teen years of three daughters, not only did I like working with the unknown, but also I had some skills transferrable to this new health crisis on the block.

The uncertainty of HIV: its relentless reign

In the 1980s and pre-1998 illness reigned relentless: Karposi's sarcoma, neuropathy, cytomegalovirus, TB, AIDS dementia, death, death and more death. HIV was in a cloud of fear, suspicion, double gloving, with don't touch, hospices and end-of-life care facilities not providing care for people who were dying.

On the other side of the coin there were committed clinicians who listened, researchers who engaged and the budding peer support movement, which was also present throughout this time. At last came the breakthrough in treatment, the Lazarus effect, as one woman described it, as she rose from the dead. There was energy, determination and of course the unrepeatable bad taste jokes.

The HIV landscape in rural Hertfordshire was mainly, but not exclusively, white gay men. In London, people from Africa were to the fore. HIV was often well down their list of immediate concerns, housing, asylum, welfare rights, safety being key.

Many African women who came to Positively Women had settled immigration status in the UK, but some had fled war or economic deprivation and were applying for asylum in the UK. Many had professional or academic backgrounds and many had held responsible positions in their country of origin, but they were not permitted to work, and if their asylum application was rejected they did not qualify for any form of financial support. Fear of people from their home country knowing of their HIV status was overwhelming. Secrecy made for vulnerability, ill health and poverty. Loss of family members from HIV, trauma, grief and fear were crushing but common experiences.

'These health tourists': colonialism alive and flourishing

I knew that destitute women were referred to the Red Cross for emergency funding. I knew women rode the night buses because they had no accommodation, that women were exploited for sex, servitude or as cheap labour in return for 'protection', somewhere to live or the keeping of their secret HIV shame. How could it be that in a wealthy country the vulnerable had to turn to the Red Cross for assistance, as if war were raging? How could people who had escaped war – 'We ran at night to escape the soldiers' – be reduced to begging? Colonialism was alive and flourishing and demeaning in action and language: 'these health tourists' 'promiscuous Africans' and most insulting, 'them'.

There was plenty more to rage about. Secrecy, shame and fear of having to pay for healthcare – and yes, people were billed for accessing healthcare – led women and men to get HIV treatment late. People were deported to their country of origin if it was designated 'safe', but where there was no HIV treatment and where they would probably die.

Decisions were made by the state that worked against good health or access to treatment. It promoted the spread of HIV and increased stigma and secrecy.

As HIV treatments became successful, I was aware that treatment research often lacked a meaningful cohort of women, let alone black women. Campaigning for this to change started by asking two 'innocent' questions at all research presentations: How many women participated in this research? Typical response: Um, none or not many. What relevance does this have for women and African women in particular? This usually brought silence.

Things have changed in clinical research; the social research on the experiences of African women and men with HIV encouraged participants to be confident, to give life stories validity and to take opportunities to have a say in HIV issues and beyond.

The strength and resilience that grew among those sharing their HIV secret, in time spilled out into the light of openness and power. In the 2000s, a young woman with HIV told me 'We are a different generation; we didn't have the struggle.'

Rage and anger are useful motivators in achieving changes, but you need to know that you are not alone in any struggle you undertake. Welcoming me to my role of CEO at Positively Women was a card from women at the support group it said, 'We can do it!'

Reflecting on the highs and lows of being part of the HIV sector

Within organisations, the endless fundraising and justifying the need for services, rising infections, people becoming ill by delaying getting tested and treatment have been some of the lows I have experienced. Parents who had rejected their sick and dying sons or daughters, because of their sexuality or HIV diagnosis, then appeared at their funerals. They had refused to hold their child's hand, speak love, comfort, reassurance in their last hours.

Some of the highlights have been working with brave and committed colleagues from 14 countries speaking a total of 23 languages and being able to support people from many African countries; and winning right to remain for many asylum seekers. I have also witnessed huge advances in treatment and care and seen activism, advocacy and visibility growing through structured peer work.

Some soundbites from life in the pressure cooker

My commitment to justice, equality and human rights was shaped by growing up in apartheid South Africa. I arrived in England with £40 and a suitcase, accepting I could not return until all citizens had the vote. Twenty-seven years later I returned for voting day. I have always lived in hope and the belief that what is right will triumph ultimately, maybe not in my lifetime, but change is possible.

Magic happens when someone has been to a peer support meeting. Peer mentoring and support looks like magic happening, but it involves rigorous training and a theoretical basis. It should be widely available and acknowledged.

Valued member of staff 10 minutes before I leave for a break:

VMS: Just one small thing to ask before you go on holiday.

Me: I will be dead and you will be knocking on my coffin with questions.

VMS: Yes and I will expect an answer.

Magazine journalist to valued member of staff:

What did you do to have HIV?

VMS: Nothing that you haven't done.

End of interview

Colleague after six years of travelling together for the European project:

Him, an anxious traveller: Elisabeth you have arrived at the right airport, at the right time, with the right luggage for the first time in six years.

Me: A triumph and an exaggeration.

Same colleague finding me after I wandered off in Berlin airport:

Elisabeth you didn't even know you were lost.

Me: Not lost, just somewhere else.

This of course, can be a good thing and is the material for miracle working.

I ended my official time in the HIV sector with a celebration that involved a performance by my daughter's light show and juggling company:

Her: What words would you like to appear in the show? I thought about, 'Fuck off you've worn me out.'

Me: Well it isn't totally true, so how about passion and pleasure?

So, passion and pleasure it was, on that night and always.

We do not learn through ease and comfort. In every problem there is a gift.

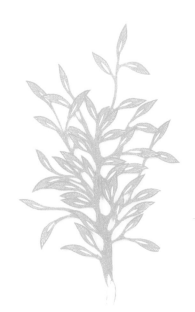

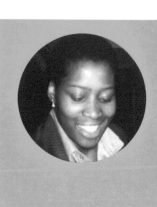

AN ACCIDENTAL HIV ACTIVIST: SCIENCE, RESEARCH AND ENSURING REPRESENTATION

Ibi Fakoya

After I finished my undergraduate degree, I knew I could never be a lab scientist. I'd spent over 100 hours in the lab spilling, forgetting-to-check, sneezing-on, dropping-down-the-sink, dropping-on-the-floor, over-exposing, under-exposing, and all-around torturing myself to clone a gene that might – just might – regulate physical stress in plants. As much as I enjoyed plant cell biology and believed that biotechnology was the key to solving global warming, I was just too clumsy for the meticulous laboratory procedures in the mid-1990s.

I decided to take a break from science. I took a job as a data entry clerk in an academic publishing company and went to evening classes to learn graphic design. After a year, I moved to the company's in-house design studio and taught myself web design, computer-generated animation and basic programming.

I had a great time working in the design studio, but at heart I was still interested in science and determined to contribute to solving the increasingly urgent problem of climate change. 'People don't care about plants,' I said to myself, 'but they do care about other people.' It's the kind of conclusion you reach when you're still too young to know how much you don't know about the world. I applied for another course – an MSc in Environmental Epidemiology and Policy at the London School of Hygiene and Tropical Medicine. If I could use science to show people that climate change will harm human health, surely governments and people would act?

Before I even finished the course, I knew two things. First, people care as much about other people as they care about plants. Pointing out the catastrophic impact of climate change on human health is not enough to provoke the urgent action needed. Second, I could contribute to something almost as important – fighting HIV and AIDS.

In September 2001, I started volunteering with the newly launched African HIV Research Forum (AHRF), co-founded by (among others) Dr Kevin Fenton and my brother Dr Ade Fakoya. The AHRF was formed in response to the rising numbers of Black African men and women diagnosed with HIV in the UK. Very little research was available about this population's HIV testing, treatment and care needs. Funding for HIV prevention was mainly geared towards men who have sex with men (MSM), as it was assumed that most HIV infections among heterosexuals were acquired in sub–Saharan Africa. It was also often assumed that black men living with HIV were heterosexual, and there was limited HIV prevention targeted at black MSM. Basically, policy-makers, healthcare commissioners, providers and others were deciding how to control the HIV epidemic in the UK in an evidence vacuum. The AHRF was there to change all that.

The AHRF was a network of researchers and practitioners who wanted to improve the development, transfer and dissemination of evidence-based practice and research in HIV and sexual health involving African communities in the UK. At first, it was run by the volunteers on the steering committee, but in 2002 funding became available for a Research Administrator/Assistant post at University College London. The post-holder would be responsible for running a new African Communities HIV Research Programme, which would be home to the AHRF. I jumped at the chance to get stuck in full time, and after a challenging interview I was appointed.

Ensuing meaningful engagement in research

Although running the research programme included a range of duties, my main interest was developing the AHRF and ensuring that people living with HIV were always meaningfully involved in research. The AHRF had clear objectives:

1. To support a strategic and ethical approach to HIV and sexual health research involving African communities in the UK
2. To establish research priorities for all areas of HIV and sexual health research with African people in the UK, including:
   - health services research
   - psychosocial research

- biomedical research

3. To facilitate implementation of research findings

4. To lead on information exchange on HIV research and knowledge transfer between healthcare workers, policy-makers, researchers and African people living with HIV

5. To collate and disseminate information about research funding opportunities

6. To increase engagement and participation of people who identify as Africans (as well as their communities) throughout the research process

7. To increase research capacity among HIV, sexual health and African communities, including Africans living with and affected by HIV.

Looking back at those objectives, it is hard to say how much we achieved. The AHRF ran from 2001 until 2011, although we were most active between 2003 and 2009. During those seven years, we organised eight seminar days, each attended by at least 80 people. The seminar days were almost festive affairs, with people from all over the country coming together to listen to the latest research, network, forge alliances and think strategically about how to ensure that Africans living in the UK were included in HIV policy, practice and research. On 7th May 2003, at the end of the fourth AHRF Seminar Day, we held an extraordinary session, 'Forming a Strategic Response to Adverse Media Reporting', led by international human rights activist Joseph O'Reilly. The session was in response to an escalating number of harmful and misleading articles in the press referring to 'HIV health tourism'. One journalist had been cherry-picking public health data and churning out alarming articles, putting the Department of Health and the Health Protection Agency under pressure to act. Although I am probably biased in my recollection of an event from 20 years ago, I remember the session generating a vibrant discussion, leaving people energised and determined to act collectively and collaboratively.

The AHRF seminar days were where new and emerging research findings were brought directly to those living with HIV. In 2005 at the 8th AHRF Seminar Day, to more than 120 community activists, nurses, doctors, policy-makers, commissioners, social workers and researchers, Dr Max Sesay (then Chief Executive of the African HIV Policy Network) formally launched the MAYISHA II report with a short speech that commended the efforts of researchers. He said, 'MAYISHA II is the largest study of sexual attitudes of Africans in England and as such a unique and valuable resource for all involved in HIV in the UK.' The AHRF was the natural place to launch the report.

AHRF activities were not just limited to seminar days; we also produced ten editions of the quarterly newsletter (AHRF News), a place for AHRF members to disseminate their research findings and a medium for sharing knowledge and training. We also published three annual research digests that summarised every relevant piece of HIV research published in the previous year.

Shoestring budgets, good will of volunteers and a forum that faded away

What happened to the AHRF? Unfortunately, like many activities run on a shoestring budget and with the goodwill of volunteers, the forum slowly faded away. The Department of Health indirectly funded the African Communities Research Programme. Although it appreciated the work of the AHRF, in 2005/06, it decided the programme should focus on evaluating the activities of the National African HIV Prevention Programme (NAHIP). I recall being deeply angry that they were limiting us instead of increasing our funding so we could expand and find additional staff to conduct evaluations and run the forum. It felt unfair, especially given that so much funding was driven toward organisations focused on the MSM community.

I continued to run the AHRF, but almost all my time was spent monitoring and evaluating HIV prevention interventions for NAHIP. Then, in 2009, I wrote my last evaluation report for NAHIP, choosing to start a new path. I was passionate about working on the AHRF and with the NAHIP partner organisations, but I was also disillusioned with the HIV landscape. Emerging Evidence for Treatment as Prevention indicated that 'test and treat' is probably the most effective HIV prevention intervention, and, consequently, funding opportunities were drying up. Although there were still gaps in the evidence, the trend toward increased funding for HIV prevention was reversing, especially considering the 2008 global financial crash. It seemed that, yet again, African HIV research was going to be pushed to the back burner, and I didn't see a future for me as a researcher if I continued devoting my time to the AHRF and NAHIP.

However, I wasn't exactly a rat leaving a sinking ship. Instead, my work became concentrated within more formal academic structures. I continued to be involved in several extensive HIV and sexual health studies, from systematic reviews into HIV testing among Black Africans on behalf National Institute for Health and Clinical Excellence to 'advancing Migrant Access to Health Services in Europe (aMASE)'. I was a co-investigator on an HIV testing trial (HAUS) and undertook the Gay Men's Sexual Health Survey and the MAYISHA II study 2016. By the time these studies were underway, the AHRF was effectively defunct, and there was no natural place to consult with people living with HIV about developing and delivering the research or a suitable arena for disseminating the study findings.

I no longer work in sexual and reproductive health, but I still use all the tips and tricks I learnt while running the AHRF. From trivial lessons ('Africans don't eat sandwiches!' and 'Don't schedule more than three speakers in an hour') to more profound insights about the true meaning of community participation in research. Because of my work with the AHRF, I can recognise when patients and the public are being marginalised instead of empowered. I know what it looks like when people come together to drive a research agenda. I know the steps required to link research successfully to policy, and policy to practise. I came to HIV sector by accident, stayed by design and left with knowledge that I am now using in my current research, understanding health system resilience to climate change.

Africans
don't eat
sandwiches.

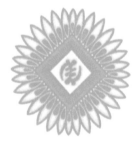

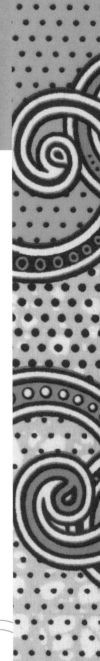

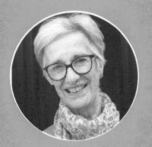

THE RIGHT PEOPLE IN THE RIGHT PLACE AT THE RIGHT TIME

Jane Anderson

It was whilst a student at St Mary's Hospital Medical School that I first heard about AIDS. I was at St Mary's because they were sympathetic to mature students, which I was, having previously studied human nutrition, and I was lucky enough to be offered a place. St Mary's was one of the first hospitals to see significant numbers of people with AIDS and was an early leader in clinical services and research. Immunologist Anthony Pinching and virologist Don Jefferies spearheaded the work and my first job as a newly qualified doctor in 1984 was working with the AIDS team.

Those early months were formative and set the course for the rest of my professional career. Under the supervision of some inspirational clinicians, I learnt about the devastating illnesses faced by people with HIV, their lives and deaths and the way others responded. I witnessed examples of the most thoughtful, innovative, brave and compassionate care, as well as fear, stigma, discrimination and abandonment. We all learnt from the people who were sick and dying, from their friends, communities, advocates and activists, and I rapidly understood that health was a political issue.

HIV care in the early days: 'I haven't seen this before'

When I first started as a new doctor 1984, HIV had only recently been discovered, with no routine testing yet available. We saw mostly young men who came into hospital very sick, and who either died on that admission or went home only to come back with new complications and dying later. There was much we didn't know, and it was a time of remarkable discovery and learning. I remember the Professor of Medicine at St Mary's coming to see a patient who had AIDS and standing at the young man's bedside, saying, 'I haven't seen this before.' It was a key experience to see one of the most knowledgeable and experienced physicians of his generation set about solving an unrecognised problem, going back to first principles of diagnosis, dealing with uncertainty and complexity. Success depended on close collaborative working with colleagues in many different departments and disciplines, some of whom were initially anxious about possible risks. I learnt early lessons in advocacy, making the case for the many tests that were needed to find out what was going on for each patient and to ensure best care.

The memories that shape you

Some of my strongest memories feature courage, bravery and activism, in particular during the early years when many people were facing appalling life-limiting illness and death. There were extraordinary responses from partners, families and friends in caring for people often in the most difficult of situations. The work of the community in bringing AIDS to public and political attention, challenging indifference and ignorance, pushing for resources and recognition have had a lasting influence on health and healthcare locally and globally.

I have also witnessed the stigma and discrimination associated with HIV with not only old, but also recent memories of people living under a cloud of fear and shame, being shockingly badly treated because of living with HIV.

Witnessing progress unfold holds many powerful memories. As better drugs became available, we got better at using them, fewer people were dying and it became apparent that effective medicines could transform dying of AIDS into living with HIV. Memories of seeing people grow older with HIV and witnessing more women with HIV confidently getting pregnant and giving birth to babies that were HIV negative and now seeing some of these children having their own children.

The unrecognised contributions of the African community to the HIV experience

Working in East London, one of the most diverse areas of the UK, I have been privileged to work very closely with African people who have backgrounds from almost every African country. Over the years the work of many of these communities in the HIV response has been under-recognised. Many are small and under-resourced, yet they have incredible energy, and their impact has been considerable. I suspect in some cases recognition has been problematic because for some communities HIV is very problematic and drawing attention to the work may be a challenge. Yet the needs of every community differ and through the work of many African community groups on HIV we have found new and innovative approaches and different ways to approach problems. It is from the experiences of people from African backgrounds in the UK that we have learnt much more about health equity and the intersectional aspects of ethnicity, gender, and migration not only in the HIV response but across the health and care system.

At a personal level, African communities have had a profound influence on my approach to medicine and healthcare. In 2000, I studied Medical Anthropology at UCL, which opened my eyes to new ways of thinking about health, medicine and wellbeing. My motivation to undertake this course of study was a direct result of working in such a diverse and exciting clinical environment with people who showed me new ways to think about healthcare and the way in which I practise medicine. Had I not met many of those women living with HIV from African communities, I wouldn't have studied and learnt more about this area that has transformed my practice.

Having a prescription pad is not enough: it's the relationships that matter

Working successfully with the complexity that surrounds HIV makes it by necessity a multidisciplinary experience, crossing organisational, professional and disciplinary boundaries. Working with so many different people and organisations has shaped my concept of what health is about, and what making a difference looks like. In particular, the joined-up working between people with lived experience and expertise and those with professional expertise is especially well developed, and in many places is a model of good practice for other areas of healthcare. HIV can be seen as the litmus paper for health and care system effectiveness; if it works for people living with and affected by HIV then it's likely to work for everyone.

HIV researcher the late Jonathan Mann was always a particularly powerful influence; we have named our clinic at Homerton for him. It was Jonathan who told us right from the beginning that HIV goes far beyond the boundaries of biological science and medicine, explaining AIDS is a political, economic and social issue and that all need to be fully addressed if HIV is to be controlled. This remains as true today as it was in Jonathan's 1987 speech to the United Nations.

Throughout my career I have worked with inspirational and dedicated clinical colleagues within the field of HIV and in other related areas. The power, expertise and dedication within the voluntary sector organisations is remarkable and an incredibly precious resource that lies behind many of the successes of the UK's HIV response. I have been fortunate to work within both the clinical and voluntary sectors, and am very proud to chair the Board of the National AIDS Trust, which has been a key influence in my life.

I've been blessed that I've met the most extraordinarily influential women in the field of HIV who have made a major difference and have taught me so much. It was a group of women at one of the World AIDS Conferences who taught me the term 'evidence-based outrage'. Without the right data and evidence, outrage is powerless, and when the evidence and data require it outrage must be the response.

Reflecting on my career highlights

Over the years there has been so much extraordinary transformational change as HIV moved from being universally fatal to a manageable condition for the long term, and it's hard to pick out particular highlights.

Helping establish the first dedicated HIV service in East London at St Bartholomew's Hospital at the start of my consultant career in 1990 was a landmark and introduced me to so many people and organisations that have had a lasting influence on my life. I believe the work we have done at Homerton in developing holistic care for people with HIV has made a difference, with social care and lived expertise from peer navigators integrated with multidisciplinary clinical care and clinical research. Securing the funding to house everything in a well-designed building that has its own garden and a labyrinth has made this a very special place. To be the Chair of the National AIDS Trust is an enormous privilege, and I am so proud of the work and impact of the organisation, and seeing London's progress within the Fast Track Cities Initiative is incredibly exciting. Ultimately, the real highlights are all the amazing people I have met along the way who have inspired me, taught me, looked after me, and allowed me to look after them. I could not have wished for a more fulfilling career.

At the heart of HIV care is a high level of engagement, partnership and collaboration. What if that could be bottled and dispensed? We could change the world.

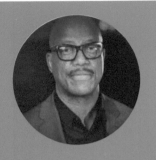

MY REFLECTIONS ON AND JOURNEY THROUGH THE HIV/AIDS PANDEMIC: A PUBLIC HEALTH PERSPECTIVE

Professor Kevin Fenton

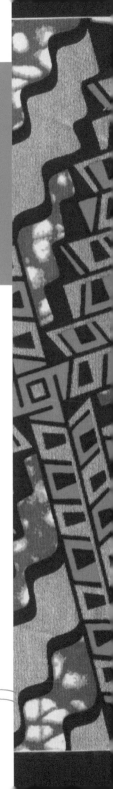

I am a British/Jamaican public health physician and infectious disease epidemiologist. I trained in Jamaica and had the privilege and opportunity to complete my postgraduate training in London in the 1990s.

I decided early in my medical training to pursue a career in public health. This was inspired by my early experiences of seeing the devastating impacts of health disparities in Jamaica, and the power of effective community health programmes, delivered at scale, to improve the health, wellbeing and life chances of millions of people.

My early clinical experiences of caring for some of the early cases of AIDS in Jamaica inspired my choice to specialise in infectious disease epidemiology with a focus on HIV/STI prevention and control.

I began training to become a physician at the beginning of the HIV/AIDS pandemic and this undoubtedly influenced my decision to work in this field and be part of finding a solution to this devastating disease. The first cases of what was then to become known as AIDS were diagnosed when I was still in high school. However, I still remember those early reports as if it were yesterday.

When I moved back to the UK in the early 1990s, before the advent of the highly effective antiretroviral treatments, I worked in clinical practice HIV and genitourinary medicine in Central London, while undertaking HIV/STI prevention research at UCL.

From the beginning of my career, I volunteered with community organisations and over the years worked closely with Big Up, Gay Men Fighting AIDS, National AIDS Trust, Terrence Higgins Trust and African HIV Policy Network. These organisations and relationships with leading HIV advocates instilled in me an understanding and respect for HIV advocacy and community-centred approaches to tackling the HIV/AIDS pandemic.

By the time I started working in the HIV sector as a clinician/researcher in the early 1990s, we already had a decade of advances in the HIV epidemic. However, many challenges remained. People were still dying from HIV in the absence of effective antiretroviral treatment, numbers of HIV infections were increasing, especially in gay and bisexual men, increasing infections, and late diagnoses and avoidable deaths were also increasing in Britain's Black African communities. There was relatively little understanding of why we were observing marked racial/ethnic differences in HIV incidence and we had very limited culturally competent HIV prevention, treatment and care programmes for our diverse communities.

On the positive side, we had the initial 1990 National Survey of Sexual Attitudes and Lifestyles (NATSAL), strong domestic and global research investments, high-quality and comprehensive clinical and supportive care for people living with HIV, good political commitment to HIV with national HIV strategies, innovative national campaigns and political engagement, a growing HIV advocacy community and a strong, integrated sexual and reproductive health services. So, a lot of work to do, and many challenges, but there was a good foundation for action and opportunities to contribute.

Sexual attitudes and beliefs: time to change the narrative creatively

Professionally, there have been so many highs over the past three decades: the availability of highly effective antiretroviral treatment, which dramatically cut deaths from AIDS; the innovative MAYISHA studies of sexual attitudes and lifestyles of Black African communities, which informed health policy and prevention programmes for Black African communities; the NATSAL II study, which studied racial/ethnic differences in sexual attitudes and lifestyles; the Department of Health and Social Care Public Health England DHSC/PHE HIV prevention innovation fund, which supported creative community prevention initiatives; the expansion of community HIV testing; and, most recently, being appointed the government's Chief HIV Advisor, charged with overseeing the implementation of the 2021 English HIV Action Plan.

I was disappointed in the delayed implementation of HIV PrEP on the NHS in England but worked closely with the DHSC and NHS England and partners to help develop the policy and approach for a national programme, leading to its eventual delivery in 2020. More generally, I am concerned about the reduction in funding to the HIV sector, especially as we are making such great gains on reducing HIV transmission; the new HIV Action Plan that will, it is hoped, ensure funding, pace and focus remains as we work to end AIDS by 2030.

Throughout my journey working on and tackling the HIV epidemic, the friendships and working relationships that I have developed along the way have been essential. My early mentors in the field, Professor Sir Michael Adler and Professor Dame Anne Johnson, provided opportunities for both high-quality training in public health and epidemiology at UCL, and encouraged me to bring my authentic self to work every day, tackling the issues that mattered to my community, which were fundamental to tackling HIV in Britain in a just and equitable way.

I am indebted to all the community advocates that I have worked with over the years for teaching me about advocacy and social justice, allowing me the space to find, understand and use my authentic voice, and to be relentless and fearless in the pursuit of health equity.

Finally, as a researcher, I have been privileged to work with so many talented and inspiring academics and public health specialists around the world that have helped improve my own scientific practice. They have opened a world of limitless possibilities in collaborating to understand why we see what we do and what we can do to improve it.

Key lessons learnt along the way

Along the way I have learnt five key life lessons that I apply to my work every day and that I share with those who I am privileged to mentor. They are:

1. Work hard. Ensure that you avail yourself of the training you need to develop the skills required for the work ahead, especially early on in your career, and do more and do better than you think you need to. Take care of your physical, mental,

emotional and spiritual health at the same time. This is non-negotiable. You can't do your best if you aren't taking care of and managing yourself well.

2. Do good work. Ensure that you align your efforts with the things that are purposeful, aligned to your values and impactful. Learn about leadership and followership, as nothing you achieve will be achieved on your own.

3. Continue to improve and learn. Life is about continued learning and improvement. Be inquisitive, collaborate, evolve and grow. Learn how to collaborate and work with others effectively, you will go further, faster and the journey will be much more fulfilling.

4. Celebrate your successes. Recognise that the journey is hard and long, and take time to celebrate and thank those who are alongside you on your journey. Practise gratitude. Pause and reflect, and remember the small positive steps for when times get hard. Every day is a new day to learn, make a difference and celebrate.

5. Give back and pay it forward. It is never too early to pay forward or to give back. Mentor, coach and support the next generation, your peers and those close to you in need. Volunteer. Treat those you work with and for you with respect and love. Look for and provide opportunities to create environments of giving, support and empowerment of others.

Towards a future that eradicated HIV: A person-centred global approach

Regarding the HIV response in the UK, I think that we are now truly on the final stage of being able to end HIV transmission by 2030. We have the tools, the will, the partnerships and the political support to do so, and the next decade should enable a resolute focus on this objective. Ending HIV transmission will be challenging because, as incidences reduce, there is a danger that the issue will fall from the policy prioritisation list and political agenda, with consequent implications for funding support, service delivery and community infrastructures. Looking to the future, a number of prerequisites for success are clear and include:

● Strategy. To enable clarity of focus and the greatest efficiency of our efforts, we need to align our actions and resources to a strategy for ending HIV transmission. The new HIV plan in England does this and must be kept under regular review.

● Stigma. This remains the last bastion of barriers to effective HIV prevention and control and now we need resolute programmes and policies to end HIV stigma in the community and in care settings. This must be coupled with continued support for education and awareness about HIV and a commitment to culturally competent approaches to tackle different forms of stigma in various communities.

- Funding support. Finding undiagnosed HIV will become more challenging as incidences reduce and strategies to promote integrated sexual health screening and opt-out HIV testing, in highest risk settings and communities, will be increasingly important.

- Global HIV control. Infectious disease knows no borders and we must continue our work to support the strategies, approaches and interventions abroad that have helped the UK to end HIV transmission, and to learn from other countries and other experiences as we progress along our elimination journey, too.

- Person-centred approaches. As we have learnt throughout the HIV pandemic, we must resist the temptation to view our efforts as only focused on the virus, but reflect and respond to the needs, opportunities and hopes of the person(s) living with the virus. The HIV pandemic taught us all about compassion, empowerment, engagement and advocacy, and these lessons will be invaluable as we make progress in reducing HIV transmission.

My top ten contributions and achievements within the field of HIV care

1. Principle co-investigator of the MAYISHA II study of sexual attitudes and lifestyles in Black African Communities in England, the first study of its kind in the UK, which helped shape national HIV policy.

2. Co-investigator on the National Survey of Sexual Attitudes and Lifestyles (NATSAL II) and lead for the survey's ethnic minority boost, which informed national and London HIV/STI prevention policy and programmes.

3. My UCL PhD theses on the epidemiology and determinants of racial/ethnic disparities in the epidemiology of HIV/STI infections in England.

4. Lead at the Health Protection Agency in England's HIV/STI Surveillance Department and lead for the Behavioural Surveillance Unit, which supported innovation in understanding behavioural trends in England.

5. Co-Principal Investigator and lead on the Gonorrhoea Resistance to Antimicrobial Surveillance Project (GRASP) in England, which informed treatment protocols for gonorrhoea.

6. Lead for ESSTI, the first European Surveillance of STI programmes, which informed the delivery of the European Centres for Disease Prevention and Control STI Surveillance programme.

7. As National Director for the US Centers for Disease Control and Prevention HIV, Viral Hepatitis, STD and TB Prevention programmes, leading on the domestic and global programme for nearly a decade.

8. Chief HIV, Sexual and Reproductive Health Advisor for Public Health England, overseeing PHE programmes for these conditions including HIV testing, the HIV innovation fund, and the foundational work for HIV PrEP in England.

9. Co-Chair of the Mayor of London's HIV Fast Track Cities Initiative, leading the multisectoral approach to ending HIV transmission and stigma and improving high-quality care in the region.

10. Being appointed Chief HIV Advisor to the Department of Health and Social Care, overseeing the implementation of the new English HIV Action Plan and Chairing the HIV Action Plan Implementation Steering Group.

The HIV and Covid-19 global pandemics have taught us that injustice anywhere results in injustice everywhere.

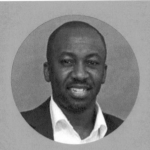

FROM LONDON TO MALAWI: CARING FOR COMMUNITIES AFFECTED BY HIV

Mas Chaponda

I went to medical school at University College London (UCL), then to a college of medicine in Malawi. That's where HIV came in. It was in the 1990s. If you can imagine Africa at that time, there were a lot of people with HIV on the wards. That was my daily life, providing care for people living with HIV. I also had lots of family members affected by HIV.

My early years as a Senior House Officer was all HIV work. All the medical wards were full of people diagnosed with HIV at varying stages of their disease journey. I was managing HIV from the word go. It was natural for me to learn about HIV as we had no treatments, and then when treatment did come along it was bit by bit.

Patients were presenting with very advanced disease, such as like cryptococcal meningitis, PCP, chronic diarrhoea, Karposi's sarcoma and lots of TB. The majority of our patients had TB, meningitis and chronic diarrhoea. We treated people the best as we could, and then gradually, probably around 1998/99, people were able to start paying for treatment. It wasn't until about 2000 that treatments were more readily available, but even then it was mainly paid-for treatment.

We were seeing a lot of people dying on a daily basis. In my own family, my uncles and my cousins died, my best friend died and my classmates died. In the wards, we were very open about it. I think there's more stigma in the UK than there was in Africa. Everybody knew about HIV and AIDS. Kenneth Kaunda, President of Zambia, talked about his son dying, which really helped people speak openly about HIV.

When I was working in the UK, I decided to go back and work in Africa and do a PhD programme (a study clinic where I started 1,000 patients on treatment). I was flying back and forth. During the time that I was there, I noticed the differences in treatments and new options available. When I was in the UK everybody was on treatment, but when I flew back to Africa only a handful of people were on treatment. We were also using Nevirpine, and I saw a lot of people experiencing hypersensitivity reactions.

I was fortunate enough to work with the eminent HIV consultant Ed Wilkins in Manchester. During that time I saw a lot of people who had survived the 1990s and were doing really well on treatment. Some of the biggest highs to this day are when I fly back home to Malawi and see people who started their journey back then and they're doing fine.

Learning from the people we provide care for

Throughout my career I have been fortunate to develop a number of meaningful relationships with my patients. I remember when I first met Craig, there was complete distrust. He looked at me, and said, 'You are going to be my doctor?' then 'When did you graduate?' He went on to ask, 'Have you treated someone like me before?' He didn't believe me when I said he would be fine. He is fine now, and he said to me the other week, 'Do you remember what I said to you when we first met?' He's such a good person, a good friend. I made lots of friends in Manchester and Liverpool.

When I worked in Manchester, very quickly I learnt from Ed and others how to inject Newfill in people who had lipodystrophy. I became friends with lots of patients, because it was such a small community then.

BHIVA has been fantastic for meeting doctors who have now become friends. I pick up the phone when I have a problem and we talk about it. I call and ask, 'What would you do with this?' and everyone jumps to help. With the pharma companies, I have found them very useful for education. At times, when I couldn't afford it, they were able to support me to go to conferences, including international ones, and I learnt a lot from this and by going on courses, including American ones. I really appreciate that exposure.

I have seen the transformation in people who were very quiet, even in clinic in the UK, sitting at the back, and during consultations almost waiting for me to talk, rather than being able to just come in and say, 'Hey, this is wrong with me' or 'I want to know more about an issue.' I've seen them became more open and started to ask questions. This has been one of my highlights. Watching people change over the years, as they've come out and become active advocates, has been fantastic.

The other thing that I've seen change in the UK is the anger some patients from the African community have felt towards social injustice and stigma. It's taken years in some cases, but I've seen a growing acceptance of the contribution made by those who have come forward and been able to talk with their family and even to others newly diagnosed.

A fellow African said to me, 'You know, when I was diagnosed, remember, you referred me to somebody who was positive, and it was fine. It was absolutely fine. It was very good, actually. I'm glad I went through that, because I now know the difference. If I sit down with another African person, the way I will relate to him will be different, because I know what questions he has in his mind that somebody from a different culture doesn't understand.'

It has been great working with Sahir House in Liverpool and the amazing people there who have given such support to the BAME (black, Asian and minority ethnic) community. There was one patient who had been in the ward for about a month. When she came to the clinic, one of the nurses said to me, 'Oh, this patient doesn't want to see you.' I thought, my god, what have I done? But then I thought OK, that's absolutely fine. We were discussing it at the end of the clinic, and I asked how the patient was. The nurse said she was fine, but very closed up, reserved: 'And you know, she doesn't want to see you.' As we left, one of the other nurses said to me, 'Do you mind if I talk to her?' I thought, feel free. The next thing I knew, I was being asked to see her in the clinic. When I saw her, I realised we were both from Malawi, and she feared I would tell everyone there. Once we connected, that was it; she didn't want to see anyone else. We laugh about it now.

What have we learnt

From a Black African perspective, I think we have learnt that the biggest problem by far is fear and stigma. HIV itself is easy. We have very good treatments, people live well and with good quality of life. So, in terms of the stigma, we need to be talking more, we need to be educating people who are young, in schools. My whole family, all my daughters, they all know. They're young, but they know about HIV. If somebody tells you that they have HIV then you should talk to them normally, laugh, joke, anything.

My priority in my life now is to make HIV treatment accessible to more people. I feel we're almost there in the UK as most diagnosed people have access to treatment. The disparity in other parts of the world is mind-blowing. I made the decision that I wanted to move and to try and focus on where the UNAIDS 95-95-95 goals are not doing so well. If you look at stigma in the Middle East, Africa and Asia, it's a really big issue. I hope in my own way I can contribute through having open conversations whilst at the same time being culturally sensitive.

The story is not over. We need to close the gap in the African HIV care experience.

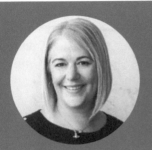

'AIDS: DON'T DIE OF IGNORANCE': THE STORIES THAT SHAPE YOU

Michelle Croston

When I was at university training to become a nurse, I worked as a healthcare support worker to get extra money and also for the experience of basic nursing care. I was always really interested in people and the stories they shared, and during this time I met a young street homeless man. Every shift he seemed to gravitate towards me, and we would have a laugh and share stories about what we were watching on TV. During these interactions he would share insights into his life and what had led him to use drugs and self-harm. This was the first time I had ever come across self-harm, so I was curious and wanted to learn more. I really enjoyed spending time with him and often lent him a comb I had that most healthcare support workers at the time carried in their pocket to help with personal care.

I remember coming on to a shift and the ward sister, someone I really admired and looked up to, pulled me to one side and said I should stop spending time with him as the doctors thought he had AIDS. I didn't know what that meant, so asked her why, as I asked my mind flashed back to the sign at the bus stop saying 'AIDS: Don't Die of Ignorance.' I was thinking to myself, that will be me, I'll die of ignorance as I don't know what it means. As if she was reading my mind the ward sister interrupted my thinking by saying, 'Because you'll catch AIDS, that's why.'

I nervously approached the patient's room and I can still see him in my mind's eye sitting on the bed looking at the floor. I asked him if he was OK and if he needed anything. As I approached him I remember him physically moving to the very end of the bed and looking scared. I wasn't sure what was happening and he said that he didn't want me to catch anything. I remember feeling sacred and confused. I'm not really sure what I said if anything. I would like to think the 18-year-old me said something kind and reassuring.

Stigma is not about knowledge

After my shift I went to the postgraduate centre to learn more about AIDS. By this time I was convinced I had given AIDS to half the ward as I had lent a few patients my comb. Hours passed in the postgraduate centre as I read more and photocopied information. This was before the internet was so freely accessible and before we had access to electronic journals, so I had to manually research all these terms and words I didn't understand. I think I drove the library staff mad with my requests.

I left the library feeling somewhat more informed, with a file thick of information, and headed up to the ward to reassure my patient and give him numbers to phone etc. Plus, I wanted to let the staff know what I had found out and I thought it was really important. When I arrived on the ward, I went into the patient's room and he had gone. I asked the night staff where he was, and they told me he had self-discharged and I sensed their relief. I tried to share the information I had found, and they just didn't seem interested. The sister I had once admired looked so unimpressed and was judgemental, which is probably the first time that I really witnessed HIV stigma.

I left the ward that night with a flea in my ear of the sister for 'getting too involved' and feeling really upset – the feeling you have when you are not 100% sure what you have done wrong mixed with a sense of injustice and a large dose of regret that I had been unable to provide the care that my patient had deserved.

Ever since that incident I have been passionate about this area of care. It was the hook that drew me in.

The HIV treatment revolution

I joined HIV care on the cusp of treatment, so I remember when I first started in the role, learning about the different combinations of drugs and dispensing very complicated regimes. Protease inhibitors were the new kids on the block and patients seemed to be responding well to treatment. As a ward-based nurse at the time, I started to see more patients leaving the ward and not returning, which was amazing. I think what I hadn't realised at the time was the psychosocial impact of HIV; that came much later in my career. I was very aware of the stigma and the impact of this on people living with HIV, but I honestly don't think I fully grasped the psychological issues people faced.

The highlights in my career have been the advances in HIV medical treatment, which has given healthcare time to explore and focus on quality of life. I think in the early days I was less aware of the psychological issues and the impact on mental health that I am now. I would also like to have focused more on women's health in the role of NHIVNA chair. I think I was so busy focusing on psychological care that I missed an opportunity to also improve outcomes for women.

I think one of my lowest moments during my career was sitting with a young pregnant woman as her two-year-old daughter was diagnosed with HIV. I think as my daughter was of a similar age my ability to connect with the situation outweighed my ability to be objective. As we were on the cusp of treatment, I was so concerned about the longer term health needs and what this would mean for the family. I could see that old ward sister shaking her head at me and warning me not to get 'too involved' – not that I have ever listened to that advice.

The importance of role models

Throughout my career people living with HIV have always been my greatest teachers. I have also really valued my relationship with Angelina Namiba and Robert Fieldhouse especially when I was chair of NHIVNA. I valued and respected their honest feedback and steer in the right direction. I have also had some really good mentors, such as great nurses Jane Bruton and Eileen Nixon, to inspire me to be a better nurse and also to show me what excellence looks like.

I think my main achievements were during my tenure as chair of NHIVNA. As an organisation, we started to shape the HIV care landscape and bring psychological care and quality of life back into the forefront of care.

I have also led on several projects that have been designed to improve outcomes for people living with HIV, annual health review, psychological care audit, review of the standards, two books and a number of research projects.

Words have the power to make or break someone, so choose them wisely.

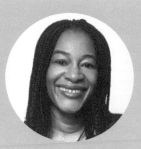

THE JOY OF WORKING IN HIV AND THE PEOPLE YOU MEET ALONG THE WAY

Nneka Nwokolo

My ending up in HIV care took a somewhat convoluted route in the sense that many things happened in my life before I joined the HIV sector, and when I made the decision to study medicine, I had virtually no knowledge of HIV.

I was born in Nigeria, but moved to Australia with my parents when I was six months old. When I was five, we moved to Papua New Guinea (PNG), where my father had taken a job teaching in the Law Faculty at the University of Papua New Guinea. Just before I turned 13, my father felt it was time for me (and later on, my siblings) to go back to Nigeria to meet his family and learn his language, so I was sent to boarding school in Onitsha, a market town in Eastern Nigeria, following which I gained entry to the University of Nigeria to study Medicine. I then moved back to PNG to complete my studies, because my parents were still there.

Having finished medical school, I did a research job with an Infectious Diseases professor from Oxford University, who, at the end of this asked if I'd like to go to the UK. I responded 'Yes', so at the end of 1993 I experienced a UK winter for the first time.

After completing my training rotations, I eventually I decided that I wanted to specialise in Infectious Diseases. I was really fascinated by HIV, so I applied to the Chelsea and Westminster Hospital HIV training rotation, got a job, and my HIV journey began.

What I loved about HIV care as I began my training was the medicine obviously, because it was interesting; but this was also a time when people were still dying, and although it was a really horrible time because of that, this was 1996/97, so the forerunners of the highly effective HIV treatments that are available today were just starting to emerge. Although it was a miserable time, from the point of view of the numbers of people dying, things soon started to change, and later it was actually a joyful time. When I started working at Chelsea, we had two wards full of people dying, Thomas Macaulay ward, which is probably the most famous of the HIV wards, and Elizabeth Gaskell Ward. People were dying, young people; it was really awful.

Within 18 months of my starting my job at Chelsea, Elizabeth Gaskell Ward closed. This left only Thomas Macaulay ward open. People didn't need to be admitted anymore, and they weren't dying as much. The reason that I would say it was joyful for me, is that it was just incredible that everybody had the same goal; we all worked together. We were all trying to do our best in the face of increasingly effective treatments, but with terrible side effects that caused awful misery. What we wanted to do was to make people's lives better, and to help people who were dying to have a good death in the best sense of the word. I think and hope that for most people we achieved this.

The friendships I have made along the way

I think the highs for me have been the friendships I've made as a result of my career in HIV. Friendships with colleagues, but also friendships with patients still alive whom I've known since my training days. When I first met them, we thought they wouldn't still be here; we thought they were going to die. I'm still very good friends with many of my colleagues who I started working with in HIV. We keep in contact, I think, because we have the memory of how we began.

The doctor–patient relationships that were created have been a source of great learning for me: learning about how to cope with really horrible situations and to overcome them; and the resilience that often people didn't know that they had. I often say in a consultation with a person who's just been diagnosed and really at their lowest, 'I know it's really bad now, but honestly, we will sit in this room together; you'll be in this chair in a year, and I promise you it will be different. Over the course of the months that lead up to that year we will meet often to review how you are doing.'

What sticks with me is the fact that people can come through circumstances that I think for many people are unimaginable. They find within themselves resources to cope and to thrive. I say this knowing that not everybody can do this, and that there are , many challenges that people face, and I'm aware that people deal with situations differently, but I have learnt so much about resilience, and so much about perspective, as a result of the relationships that I have made.

The evolving world of HIV knowledge, treatment and care

Knowledge and understanding of HIV have evolved and increased over the last 40 years in a way that I think has not been the case for many diseases areas. It's a real testament to the fact that if you have engagement and enough interest, and you have people to drive things, this is what can happen. Which is also unfortunate, as well, and I think brings with it a lesson, which is that if you can do this for HIV, because of some people's activism, why can it not be done for other conditions that have been around for a long time, that affect people who are not perceived as being as important?

One of the lows for me came when antiretroviral therapy was rolled out in the west and was not available in Africa. The conversations that were happening at that time were, you know, were words to the effect that, 'Oh, you can't have antiretroviral therapy in Africa, because they won't take it properly. It's too expensive. We should be focusing on prevention in Africa, not treatment.'

Activism at it best

The lack of antiretroviral therapy led to the huge activism in the UK from organisations such as the AHPN, some of which don't necessarily exist anymore. The engagement and the conversations with these early groups of African activists raised the profile of HIV within the African community, but also externally. At that time, the two groups of people who are most affected by HIV were predominantly white men who have sex with men, and Africans. There was, unfortunately, the narrative at the time was that these two groups of people were basically bringers and harbingers of disease. The conversation was really negative. The work that organisations like the AHPN did to try to counter that narrative successfully was so important. They were the driving forces behind how far we've come in our understanding of HIV. It's a testament to the work of these early pioneers, African pioneers, that so many people are on treatment, that so many people are testing, that we know about U=U, that we know about treatment as prevention, and all of that is down to the work of those organisations and activists.

In the UK, there is still a lot of work to be done with regard to updating the general public on where HIV is now. The fact that HIV is not talked about very much in the general public because it's not perceived as being a problem can be seen as a negative in one way. It can also be seen as a positive, because of all that negativity and the depths of misconception that still exist based on a time before the advances in treatment that exist now, and our current understanding of HIV care. We do have to make sure that in the general population understand that HIV is still a thing, and that it can affect anyone.

Creating a culture that looks out for each other

Within the third sector, there's a lot of competition for funds and that often creates a situation where the organisations that provide funding, whether they do it deliberately or not, pit organisations against each other, which is so wrong, because we all want the same thing. What ends up happening is that big organisations tend to be seen as more successful, more useful, than smaller organisations. Some of the big organisations can be at an advantage because they have departments or people dedicated to writing funding bids, and smaller organisations don't have that. It could be argued that potentially smaller organisations are closer to the people who need this help than the big organisations. We should try really hard as a community to stop this, to find a way to have an umbrella under which everybody who is trying to reach the same goal can do so together.

When I reflect on my career, I am really proud of what I see as my advocacy for women living with HIV, and women in general. I want to find ways to keep that going for as long as I'm alive, because it is really important to me, the work that I'm trying to do to help tackle stigma related to HIV in the general population, and also now with my work relating to older women and menopause and the stigma associated with that.

We need to have an umbrella organisation that receives funding, then shares this funding with other organisations to support people to keep them safe.

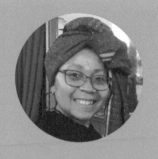

THE BLACK COMMUNITY NEEDS A VOICE: AN INTOXICATING MIX OF ANGER, PASSION, HOPE AND DESIRE

Priscilla Nkwenti

I came to England in October 1982 from Cameroon. I had never heard of GRID (Gay-Related Immune Deficiency) or AIDS. I was brought up in a Christian household and my parents were church elders, visiting the sick and sharing what they had with those who had very little compared to them. Their values were directly instilled in me and my siblings. I also attended an all-girls boarding secondary school for five years and during that time I joined various clubs that recruited volunteers to go out into the community and visit the sick, fetch water and sometimes clean their homes. My volunteering years started way before I came to the UK. It was instilled in me and still is in my DNA.

I was an undergraduate student in Liverpool when I saw a poster in the student coffee room appealing for blood donors. I picked up an accompanying leaflet that explained the need for donating blood and gave dates when the blood-collecting van will be on campus. I decided to become a blood donor and turned up on the day and was registered and started my blood donation journey for three years. This came to an end in 1986 after I had moved to London and was then a postgraduate student.

The first I heard of HIV/AIDS was in 1986 when the 'AIDS: Don't Die of Ignorance' public health campaign hit the nation. Soon after, it was brought to my attention that I could no longer give blood because I had come into the UK from sub-Saharan Africa and had previously had sex with someone from that part of the world, too. My blood-donation days were truly over. However, my dormant interest in HIV/AIDS had been rudely awakened. I read avidly about HIV and its origins, and the more I read the more unsettled I became.

Following my sojourn to London, I moved back north in 1988 when I got married and settled in Manchester. I got a job with the Church of England as a Community Development Worker, which was a proxy social worker. I worked with and supported parishioners, 90% of whom were from black and minority ethnic communities. Through my work, I reached out and worked closely with organisations in the voluntary as well as the public sector, raising awareness of some of the health and social care challenges faced by the parishioners.

Whilst working for the Church of England, I attended a lot of meetings where decisions were made, and suggestions and proposals tabled and debated. I soon realised that the experiences of individuals in society had to be pivotal in decision-making, service planning, delivery and monitoring, a lesson that would prepare me for working in the world of HIV/AIDS. It would enable and provide succour when faced with the many challenges that came with working with disproportionately affected population groups.

In 1990, Manchester City Council organised a meeting to discuss the impact of HIV/AIDS in black communities. I attended the meeting and was propelled into an intoxicating mix of anger, passion, hope and the desire to fight to make things right for all individuals living with HIV/AIDS and to work with and support communities affected otherwise.

At the end of that meeting, I volunteered to join a group that was being set up, subsequently named Black HIV & AIDS Forum (BHAF). BHAF was set up initially as a pressure group to ensure black communities had access to accurate and culturally appropriate information about HIV including care and support services. I joined initially as a volunteer and then became the HIV Public Education Officer in 1991.

Whilst I was working for the Church of England, a needle exchange scheme was set up in Hulme on the doorstep of the Ascension Church where I was based. The needle exchange was an initiative of Manchester City Council to reduce the harm caused to individuals who inject drugs. Rather than share and use dirty needles, users bring the used ones to the exchange and collect new and clean ones. The scheme advised drug users not to share needles with the aim of reducing blood-borne viruses and bacterial infections. I represented the church at the needle exchange planning meetings and played a key role in explaining the need for and health benefits of the needle exchange not just to the church congregation, but also to community groups who were very concerned that used needles would be strewn all over the place.

Being drawn to work in the sector

The fear, stigma and discrimination that HIV generated at individual and societal level fuelled my own insecurities. I observed the full effects of this whilst volunteering at a needle exchange scheme. I had a desire to learn, understand and see HIV for what it really was at a sociocultural, socio-political, geopolitical and economic development level. These were the main drivers for me to become involved in this sector. I held an intrinsic believe that HIV prevention and HIV support services could and should be improved to better serve the needs of black people, both living with HIV and affected.

The old fever hospitals

Monsall Hospital was established as a hospital for fever patients in 1871 and in 1925, and became a hospital for infectious diseases. Before it closed in 1993, all individuals in Manchester and the surrounding boroughs who were diagnosed with HIV or AIDS were admitted and treated within its facilities. I remember undertaking weekly visits to the hospital to sit with very, very sick and scared service users. There was lots of whirring of equipment and very little else on the AIDS ward. The cocktail of tablets that were prescribed and ingested on a daily basis and the restrictions in relation to food and drug interactions ... it was overwhelming!

There was a lot of confusion as black people were told to eat certain western foods that they were not used to. This led to my colleagues and I cooking and taking African and Caribbean food to our service users in hospital. We also got involved in hair braiding in hospital and body moisturising after bed baths.

The eerie silence driving away from the hospital will be something that will stay with me. We also carried out a number of home visits to provide some level of emotional, as well as practical support. Asylum seekers and undocumented migrants were often too scared to access whatever little care and support was available from both the public and voluntary sector. We supported people giving up, dropping out of college or university and just waiting to die. We staffed helplines that provided advice and support, but mainly in English and culturally unaware. During this time, I attended funerals on a regular basis, with family members of the deceased insisting that the cause of death should not be stated in eulogies for fear of reprisals from the community.

The evolution of activism

It fills me with pride to see the activism that HIV and AIDS eventually generated in the African communities, most of all seeing key individuals living with HIV standing at the frontline, leading and taking the African community to heights and levels that were unthinkable 30 years ago.

Since the 1980s, there has been an increase in HIV community activists working at grassroots level leading and championing the needs of the African population groups. Seeing the number of black-led organisations that have been set up to work both with communities and with policy-makers has been a powerful moment for me.

Despite the advances we have made with our activism in these communities, there still remains ongoing fear and stigma in parts of our African community, and individuals still experience discrimination within their community. This is coupled with the ongoing and continuous reduction in funding, which can lead to partnership working not really being as productive as it could be.

An open door policy

My relationships with African organisations and community groups, including faith groups, have been profound. The group members have been insightful and knowledgeable and confident to challenge both development and delivery plans. The trust built over so many years has allowed for frank and open discussions even on very sensitive topics. Involving and engaging the communities in strategic development has meant that they have owned it and worked alongside to ensure delivery. My relationship with organisations that address the diversity within gender identity has been most enlightening. My relationship with the majority of our funders and commissioners has been commendable, which has led to strong working relationships with them. I have been honest and not withheld information even when I have faced challenges and not delivered as expected. Always working together to discuss and agree how we tackle challenges has helped. My relationship with my staff and volunteers has been close as I have been open, honest and accommodating and shown appreciation for hard work and achievements. My open door policy has helped.

Advocating for cultural appropriate HIV prevention and care

I started work in the HIV/AIDS sector in the early 1990s and worked for over 30 years raising awareness on HIV transmission and HIV prevention in the African community. I contributed to normalising conversations on sex and relationships, albeit it took a long time.

Whilst studying for my PhD, I ran a series of focus groups that brought African women together to establish barriers to condom use and the dynamics of sexual relationships with various African cultural gender norms. The findings from the focus group not only informed my research, but also contributed to the thinking behind setting up an African Women's Health Forum in Manchester.

I was instrumental in applying for and winning a national helpline contract that provided culturally appropriate and sensitive HIV prevention, treatment and care information in several African languages. The National HIV Prevention Programme enabled support of community-based organisations to integrate HIV prevention in their remit. As a member of a number of regional and national task forces, I have contributed to debates and discussions on community testing.

Throughout my career, I provided training to a range of public and voluntary sector organisations on how to integrate cultural issues in the provision of their services HIV services, which has undoubtedly improved outcomes or people living with HIV.

Take calculated risks and some not so calculated.

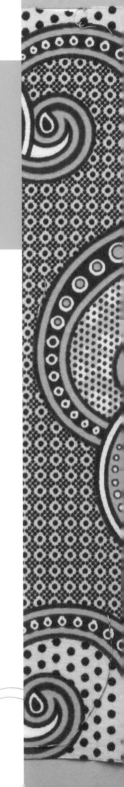

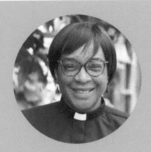

FROM A CONSERVATIVE CHRISTIAN BACKGROUND TO A WORLD OF HIV ACTIVISM AND FAITH

Rev Ije Ajibade

was born in the UK, with my two sisters. My dad was a lecturer at Norwich City College and my mum was a nurse. When I was 12 years old, the whole family moved back to Nigeria, except for my older sister who was studying nursing at the time.

In Nigeria I went to boarding school, then on to university and law school. Then the whole family came back to the UK. Unfortunately, both my parents and older sister have since passed away.

In the early 2000s, I was working at the mayor's office in London, working on scrutiny for the London Assembly. They decided to do a scrutiny of HIV services in London. This involved setting up committee hearings, which involved many HIV organisations giving evidence. Some of the organisations included the National AIDS Trust, the Terrence Higgins Trust (THT), the African HIV Policy Network, now the African Health Policy Network (AHPN), and a few others.

It is through this piece of work that I learnt a lot about HIV. I met many HIV activists, especially black women activists, and I was impressed by them. Coming from a conservative Christian background you hear a lot of disapproval and stigmatisation of people who are not heterosexual, especially against men having sex with men. After the select committee hearing on HIV, I contacted a few HIV organisations that had participated and asked them how I could support their work. I ended up on the boards of the NAZ Project London and the AHPN. I also helped the AHPN in formulating its work on HIV and faith.

Hearing the invisible voices of HIV activism

I only saw the HIV landscape through the AHPN lens when I was supporting their work. At the time I got involved, I felt there were more voices, a lot more activity, especially on HIV prevention. HIV as an issue was visible and I heard about many outreach events. I remember engaging faith leaders on HIV, but I am not sure we made the impact we wanted to make.

My experience of working with various individuals and organisations in the HIV sector enabled me to preach on HIV, especially when I became a priest and was called to minister. I initiated workshops on HIV and faith as part of educating and getting faith communities involved in HIV. I also made sure to do an annual service on World AIDS Day.

I feel people living with HIV, especially within the black communities, were empowered to speak up. They were encouraged to live their lives with dignity, openly living with HIV and being supported to lead. I also feel that there was much more HIV awareness back then in the early 2000s.

As African communities in the diaspora, we tend to be very fractured. We focus a lot on our differences and not what we have in common. However, when it came to HIV, we were forced to come together and to speak with one voice. This helped us access funding as communities, especially under the national umbrella of the AHPN organisation. I feel that this also helped us to start thinking about other issues that we could continue working on in the future.

However, then HIV was reprioritised in terms of funding at the global and country levels, and things started to wane. There was less and less HIV information and activity, to a point that when Covid-19 appeared I heard people say we have never been through anything like a pandemic.

I had to remind some people that we do have an HIV pandemic still going on, a pandemic that has killed more than 30 million people globally! It is just that it is silent, stigmatised and affecting marginalised groups. Some people have lived in a pandemic their whole lives; it is their life story.

Grappling with theology: engaging with faith leaders on HIV

Throughout my career I have amplified the voice of faith on this subject, especially as a Black African woman. I supported people to grapple with the theology and to engage faith leaders on HIV, making them understand the issues, their impact on people living with HIV and the implications for our faith communities.

Through my work with the London Assembly up to when I was ordained as a priest, I was able to preach the gospel of inclusivity, walking alongside people living with HIV and being a friend. Being there for people was very important to me.

In 2011, I attended the UN Special Session on AIDS in New York as part of my role at the AHPN. I interacted with many global HIV activists and when I got back to the UK, I remember preaching about it, as the best example of what the Feast of Pentecost represents. The Holy Spirit was working through the activists from around the world to do the work they were doing.

I still preach about HIV in my sermons. It has really shaped my faith and left such a mark on me. I worked with the World Council of Churches, contributing to sermons a publication on HIV and faith. I have also written a number of HIV articles for various organisations around the world, essays and journal publications.

When I was ordained a priest, the service took place at St Paul's Cathedral in London, and so many people working in the HIV sector attended the service. They felt that I had been there for them, and they came to support me.

I built really strong friendships with many people in the HIV sector, friendships I hold dear to this day. Many people moved on to different parts of the world, either for work or to return home to their countries, but we meet up now and then when they visit London. It is like a global HIV family that I gained when I engaged with HIV and I will treasure this family for the rest of my life.

I have been to weddings, christenings and all manner of events, in different countries to be there for friends I met in the HIV sector. There is a bible passage that talks about a friend who is closer than a brother, and that is what I got from my HIV activism, friendships and family for life.

Finding my voice as an African woman

When you are born and brought up outside your country of origin, you can lose the connections to that country and feel very rootless. Working on HIV really grounded me in the African diaspora. I had an African identity before this, but as I worked with other African activists a cultural gap was filled. Working on HIV helped me flourish and find my voice as an African woman in the UK.

The African HIV response is an example of Black Lives Matter. It was about demanding and being part of creating services that were culturally appropriate to our communities. We did it with dignity, volunteering long hours, doing outreach in our churches and communities, in an environment that was antagonistic to us as migrants as well as black people.

Whatever I learnt through working on HIV, I have carried into all the work I have done ever since. Working on challenging issues like HIV and sexuality empowered me to deal with complex human rights issues in other areas, such as the maritime industry. Working on HIV has empowered me to look more closely at the world around me and strive for justice wherever I may find myself.

HIV activism is empowering, but never easy.

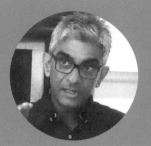

FOLLOWING A DREAM: IN PURSUIT OF A CAREER IN HIV MEDICINE

Sanjay Bhagani

I was born and brought up in Kitale on the Western border of Kenya and grew up in the idyllic coastal town of Mombasa. Whilst a student at school, I always wanted to become a doctor and was fortunate enough to be able to come to the UK to study medicine. There were no doctors in our family (my father was a businessman) and there was a huge amount of support and sacrifice from my family to enable me to follow my dream.

Whilst I was at medical school in Leicester in the mid-1980s, the first AIDS cases had just been described in the USA, and there were reports of 'slim disease' affecting people in Uganda. That was a challenge I set myself; this was the disease area I was going to specialise in and help overcome. Of course, these were big aspirations, since it was only whilst I was in second year at medical school that the virus causing AIDS was first discovered. It felt like this would be the ideal area where I could apply myself in the future. However, before that there were many years of training yet to go.

My first real involvement in HIV care didn't come until 1994 when I had completed my undergraduate and the first bit of postgraduate training in Leicester. (There were very few diagnosed people living with HIV in Leicester at the time.) I opted to specialise in infectious diseases in order to pursue a career in HIV medicine, which it wasn't (and is still not) recognised as a specialty in its own right. I came to London and was fortunate enough to start my first job in the Ian Charleston Centre at the Royal Free Hospital, where I learnt all about managing people living with HIV.

AZT had already been licensed and dual therapy was beginning to hit the limelight. Most of our care was supportive, treating and preventing opportunistic infections, symptom control and, when necessary, palliative care with dignity. I learnt a lot about how hopeless people living with HIV often felt and the stigma of HIV (which unfortunately still exists), a really difficult position both for themselves and their loved ones.

The impact of not taking treatment and the advances in science

Perhaps my low point was the mid-1990s, when as a clinician often all I could offer was a dignified, pain-free, peaceful end for many of my patients. That was really frustrating. I still feel that way sometimes when I see late presenters or patients presenting with devastating opportunistic infections because they haven't taken treatment properly.

Of course, the high point was when the first results of the triple therapy with protease inhibitors – what was called HAART in those days – were first announced. However, it took many years before we were able to see those results translate into care to change the lives of many. Perhaps the real high was when we saw the results of the PARTNER study and the concept of U=U. I sincerely hope this will change the lives of many and has a significant impact on reducing stigma.

A personal high from a career point of view was when I was appointed a Consultant in Infectious Diseases and HIV Medicine, and I could influence the way we provided care for people living with HIV in our clinic.

My relationship with my patients has been the most meaningful part of my journey so far. The need to be guided by the person in front of me, in terms of the care and support they require is a crucial aspect of clinical care that every clinician who embarks on this journey must learn.

When I took over, I was President of the European AIDS Clinical Society (EACS), I was insistent that we would strengthen our education programme so global care for people living with HIV was uniform and at the highest standard achievable. Training the next generation of healthcare providers will be crucial for our mission.

A regret that still stands is that I never went back to practise HIV medicine in East Africa, although I contribute to teaching, research and research training in the region. I hope to be able to fulfil this aspect of my aspirations in the next couple of years.

Activism and the African communities

Whilst activism was crucial in the HIV response, this was driven mostly by the hugely influential white Caucasian men who have sex with men voice in the early days. I realised from my own clinical experience that at least a third of our patients were of African origin, many here in the UK under very difficult circumstances. When African voices began to emerge in activism, support for care, rights for women living with HIV, this felt like a real turning-point for the African communities both on the African continent and abroad.

Perhaps an important lesson from the Covid-19 pandemic was that when we put our minds and resources with multinational support we can change (and influence) the course of an illness quickly. The HIV response has been slow(er); there are still many hurdles to cross, particularly in parts of sub-Saharan Africa and Eastern/Central Europe, in terms of care and access to therapy and prevention services. There are still huge hurdles to cross in terms of tackling stigma.

Apart from excellence in care for individual patients, I hope to have made a significant contribution to the field of HIV/hepatitis co-infection and teaching/training of future generation of HIV clinicians. My career is not over yet. I sincerely I hope I can continue caring for individual patients and teaching and have the opportunity to go back 'home' to provide some more direct input.

I wish for a world free from the suffering and stigma associated with HIV.

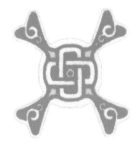

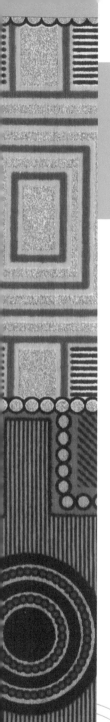

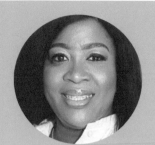

HAVING THE PRIVILEGE OF WORKING IN HIV CARE

Vanessa Apea

I was 18 when I started medical school at Guy's and St Thomas'. At the same time, I lost a close relative to cancer and decided that I wanted to specialise in oncology. Everything I did was geared towards cancer care. Then came my last job before oncology training in sexual health and HIV. I had actually decided that I wouldn't do the job, but took it as the department was short-staffed. I am so glad I did as I fell in love with the speciality.

I was first based at the Ambrose King Centre, a sexual health clinic in East London and early on I felt it was an area in which you could really make a difference. It is a unique opportunity to see someone coming into clinic, nervous and anxious, some with feelings of shame and stigma; then within minutes, you have the potential, and privilege, to reshape their feelings completely into a positive experience.

Mixed memories of the early days of working in HIV care

At this time in 2005, the HIV wards were full of people living with and dying from advanced HIV. There was a real mix of people, of varying gender, ethnicity and sexuality. Being in East London, there were many heterosexual people of African descent. We then witnessed the advent of combined antiretroviral therapy, which led to massive changes within HIV care.

The most impactful aspects for me were the patients and the staff that I worked with. So much was just so raw at that time. Watching people and their loved ones navigate HIV and all that it entailed was both inspiring and painful. Despite advances in scientific knowledge, there was just a lot of loss, unnecessary loss at that, and it was hard to watch it all unfold. Watching families have a lot of anger and confusion, in the midst of grief was immensely difficult. Often, the ones who were left behind struggled to process what had happened as they couldn't understand why they had lost their loved one in this way.

The trust that people place in us as healthcare professionals always amazes me and I view it as a huge privilege. As a doctor, people feel safe to confide in you and share truly sensitive information about themselves that they might not ordinarily share with anybody else and may even find it hard to admit to themselves. Just being able to respond with kindness and prioritise someone's care, and being able to say to them, 'Forget what society is saying, forget what your family say, forget everything else in this moment and let's concentrate on you. You're here and we're caring for you,' was often, if not always, one of the best parts of my job.

What also often struck me during this time was the relationship between the medics, nurses, physiotherapists, administrators and other healthcare professionals; we were all like one big family working together, with each patient and their family. It was a really powerful experience with everyone on the same page. Everyone was committed to providing dignity to all people living with HIV, both in life and in death.

The power of stigma

Watching stigma present itself in clinical environments and seeing the dual life that people often have to lead is always really difficult. You see people in clinic, and they're sobbing, anxious, scared and then they pick themselves up and step back out into the outside world, rarely sharing their diagnosis or lived realities with anyone. Watching people having their quality of life limited due to the ignorance and stigma that surrounds HIV saddens me and motivates me to play my role in eliminating stigma.

When supporting people to tell their loved ones about their diagnosis, we often see the manifestation of internalised stigma of the person living with HIV and the external stigma and biases experienced by them. When processing difficult things, people's first reactions and behaviour tend not be the best of responses. After telling others about their diagnosis people living with HIV may have to experience, process and move past such traumatic responses impacting on their self-esteem and self-perception.

One standout memory for me was when this assumption of a negative reaction was challenged. I remember providing care for a heterosexual married couple of Central African heritage. The wife had been diagnosed in pregnancy, just before delivery, and it was a massive whirlwind for all involved. I'll never forget that day. Our entire clinical team were certain that once the husband got the news that his wife was living with HIV, there would be an extremely negative reaction. We were on high alert, and ready to intervene come what may. When the husband was informed he listened calmly and patiently. A few days later when he was confirmed as HIV negative, he gently asked if he could have a word. He then confided in me, saying, 'I don't know what to do because she feels like I'm going to leave her. To me it doesn't matter. I love her, it's not her fault. It is no one's fault.' When I reflect on this, it serves both as a personal reminder of the need to challenge continually my own unconscious biases and as a glimpse of what life could be like without stigma and ignorance.

The people who have shaped my personal journey

I feel really honoured that I have been mentored and taught by some of the most influential people in sexual health and HIV, such as Dr Beng Goh, Professor Chloe Orkin, Dr Liat Sarner, Professor Jane Anderson, Dr Maurice Murphy and Dr Simon Rackstraw. Watching them navigate the sector and how they supported and advocated for people was so inspiring. They demonstrated what needed to be done and what should be done for all.

In addition, all the nurses, pharmacists, social workers, psychologists, health advisors, physiotherapists and occupational therapists that I have developed relationships with have been pivotal in my journey. These professional and personal relationships in which you supported each other and gave each other strength, but were also able to critique and safely reflect, am I doing this in the right way? How can I help this person more?

Then came peer mentors! Sophie Strachan was the first peer mentor in our clinic and she cultivated such impactful relationships with clinicians and people attending our clinic. She worked closely with us to create better spaces in which people could just be open and honest about who they were and what they needed. This was invaluable.

We talk more and more about representation nowadays, but the HIV sector has always led the way. I feel African communities within the HIV sector have particularly demonstrated the power of representation. Many have moved past their personal vulnerabilities and internalised and external stigma to convey their lived experience in order to support peers and educate others in the sector enabling them to provide better care. Many people in the HIV sector realise that the African communities stepped up and made the sector realise that they could not progress without them. They shone a light on groups that were missed and not often heard or prioritised. They emphasised that all communities needed to be front and centre of the response. It is clear that if many key individuals did not step up, and show people what was needed, we wouldn't have got to where we are now.

The sector would not have any inkling of the lived experience of varied African settings were it not for the HIV African communities here telling them. Many have shown what it means to be unapologetic about being African and showing the richness and pride that people have as Africans. I was born and raised in East London, but my parents are both from Ghana. A lot of my childhood involved going back and forth to Ghana and having the opportunity to step into both worlds, so much of my life in the UK is impacted by Ghanaian heritage and social networks. HIV is a globalised story and more needs to be done to recognise the power and impact of the diasporan mindset. A mindset that is shaped by what's going on back home.

On a personal level, I have found my representation as a black woman, as a black doctor, in this sector matters. I've tried to use this platform to challenge stigma, to advocate and research, with the hope that I deliver the best care possible and challenge when the people are not receiving the care they deserve.

There are always people who fall through the safety nets we create in access and care. We need to find ways to prevent this. We need to listen to people, learn from them and intentionally respond.

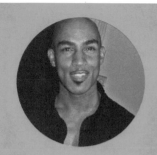

THEIR SHOES COULD FIT MY FEET: SUPPORTING REAL PEOPLE

Vernal Scott

I was born at St Mary's Hospital in 1960s London to Jamaican parents. In the mid-1980s I launched the People's (multicultural) Group at the London Lesbian & Gay Centre, and later founded the Black Communities AIDS Team. In 1987, I was appointed Head of HIV services for Brent Council, and in 2003 joined Islington Council as Head of Equality and Diversity. In 2017, I joined Havering Council as Equality lead, and in June 2020, during the worldwide Black Lives Matter protests that followed the murder of George Floyd by a serving US police officer, I joined the UK police service, in Diversity and Inclusion at Essex Police.

There was nothing more important to do with my life. As a gay man, I felt a need to support people affected by HIV and social injustice; their shoes could fit my feet. To me, they were not statistics, but real men, women and children: our loved ones, friends, lovers, children, colleagues and neighbours. Real people! This was reflected in the people I saw at the Brent HIV Centre, who included teachers, policemen, scientists, authors, artists, lawyers, performers, businesspeople, accountants, IT specialists, managers, caterers, students and health service staff. The youngest person at the centre was born to an infected mother and was just eighteen months old, and the oldest was a gay man in his late fifties. They were of different nationalities and income brackets and possessed incalculable talent, skills and accomplishments.

Booted out of your own party and what a blessing for humanity

I have been involved in HIV care since the mid-1980s. By 1991, Mrs Thatcher had been booted out by her own party, and I, for one, wasn't sad to see her go. She had been a capable Prime Minister, even if her politics and mine were worlds apart, but she lacked humanity for anyone who didn't look or sound like her, or whose lifestyle was different. We needed a human being at the helm at this time of trauma and crisis, not someone who took pride in being referred to as the Iron Lady. Norman Fowler, her by now former Secretary of State for Health, seemed more human during his tenure in the job, even if his stone-cold 'AIDS: Don't Die of Ignorance' campaign failed to convey an ounce of empathy with the bereaved and dying. He disappointed many of us further when he voted in favour of Clause 28, the UK's infamous anti-gay legislation. Our horrible deaths were not enough; we were down and being kicked by our own government, the people who would have happily taken care of us if only we had been heterosexual. There were by then between two and three million AIDS cases reported around the world. My attention remained focused on the human experience behind the mounting numbers.

Some of my greatest highs when working within HIV care include developing the Brent HIV Centre, and getting the personal support of celebrities such as Whitney Houston, George Michael and Dionne Warwick. However, this was also overshadowed by burying family members, as well as many friends, lovers and service users. It was a horrible time, but it taught me how tough I could be, emotionally and practically.

With endings come new beginnings

My lifelong relationship with God ended during my time working at the Brent HIV Centre. There was too much death and dying to continue to believe in him, which led me to write my book *God's other children – a London Memoir*. I thought over time I would get back my faith and believe in God again, but my faith remains dead. This made way for the most important relationships I developed with the service users and the friends directly affected by HIV. During this time, the black and gay communities learnt that when we have no option but to be strong, we are capable of being stronger than we ever thought possible. HIV has inflicted too much pain on so many lives. I hope one day that we will be able to end HIV stigma – Diana, Whitney and others tried to. I include HIV in our general inclusion training in the police service, but it is still a challenge.

We should continue to tap into our collective strength to build a better future. We are the drivers (not the passengers) towards the destiny of our choosing.

THIS SUMMER

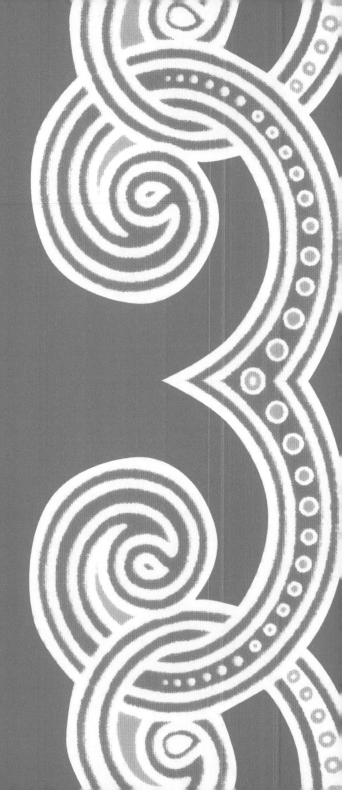

This summer, what matters is
Peace, joy, and happiness.
Me, me, me! In the nicest possible way.
Bring on the summer!
This summer I choose to live
In a space full of love, life, and laughter.
Mindfully, enthusiastically, passionately.
I will live life to the fullest, to appreciate
Every single day that I am alive.
I choose to live life at a slower pace
Packed with fun and self-love stuff.
I will sway like a tree,
And dance like the leaves,
Floating in the air.

Group poem

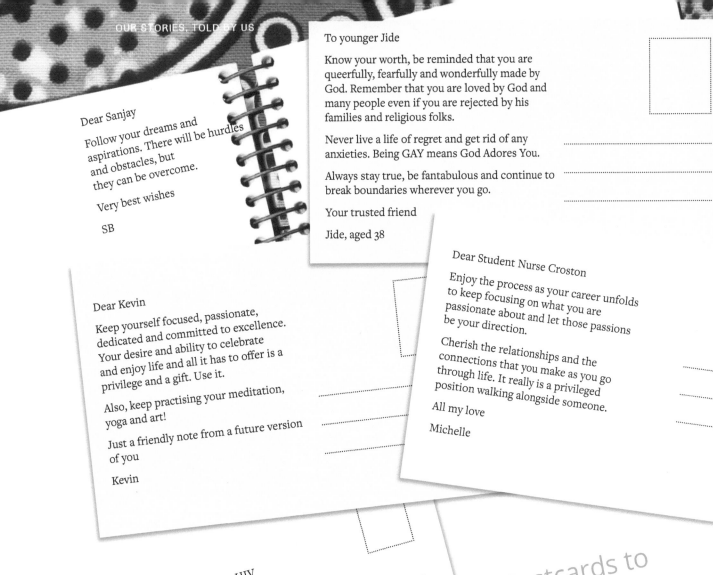

Dear Sanjay

Follow your dreams and aspirations. There will be hurdles and obstacles, but they can be overcome.

Very best wishes

SB

To younger Jide

Know your worth, be reminded that you are queerfully, fearfully and wonderfully made by God. Remember that you are loved by God and many people even if you are rejected by his families and religious folks.

Never live a life of regret and get rid of any anxieties. Being GAY means God Adores You.

Always stay true, be fantabulous and continue to break boundaries wherever you go.

Your trusted friend

Jide, aged 38

Dear Kevin

Keep yourself focused, passionate, dedicated and committed to excellence. Your desire and ability to celebrate and enjoy life and all it has to offer is a privilege and a gift. Use it.

Also, keep practising your meditation, yoga and art!

Just a friendly note from a future version of you

Kevin

Dear Student Nurse Croston

Enjoy the process as your career unfolds to keep focusing on what you are passionate about and let those passions be your direction.

Cherish the relationships and the connections that you make as you go through life. It really is a privileged position walking alongside someone.

All my love

Michelle

Future Bakita

Take breaks. Take a break out of the HIV sector where necessary. You don't need to do it all and you do need to take breaks. You've had a few, and you know that you've burnt out a few times. Last year was the worst to date.

Let's not have a repeat performance.

B

Postcards to a different version of me

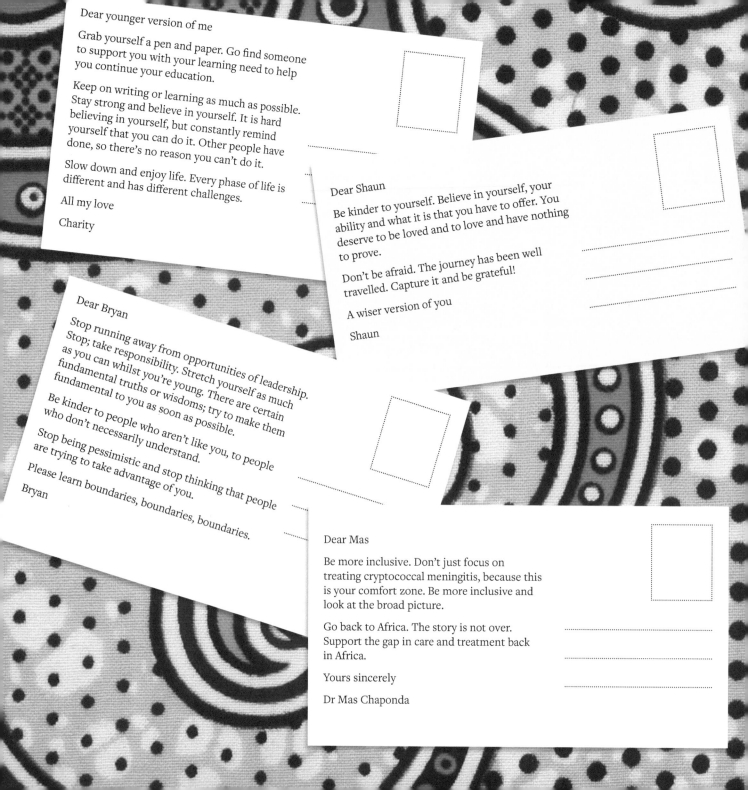

Dear younger version of me

Grab yourself a pen and paper. Go find someone to support you with your learning need to help you continue your education.

Keep on writing or learning as much as possible. Stay strong and believe in yourself. It is hard believing in yourself, but constantly remind yourself that you can do it. Other people have done, so there's no reason you can't do it.

Slow down and enjoy life. Every phase of life is different and has different challenges.

All my love

Charity

Dear Shaun

Be kinder to yourself. Believe in yourself, your ability and what it is that you have to offer. You deserve to be loved and to love and have nothing to prove.

Don't be afraid. The journey has been well travelled. Capture it and be grateful!

A wiser version of you

Shaun

Dear Bryan

Stop running away from opportunities of leadership. Stop; take responsibility. Stretch yourself as much as you can whilst you're young. There are certain fundamental truths or wisdoms; try to make them fundamental to you as soon as possible.

Be kinder to people who aren't like you, to people who don't necessarily understand.

Stop being pessimistic and stop thinking that people are trying to take advantage of you.

Please learn boundaries, boundaries, boundaries.

Bryan

Dear Mas

Be more inclusive. Don't just focus on treating cryptococcal meningitis, because this is your comfort zone. Be more inclusive and look at the broad picture.

Go back to Africa. The story is not over. Support the gap in care and treatment back in Africa.

Yours sincerely

Dr Mas Chaponda

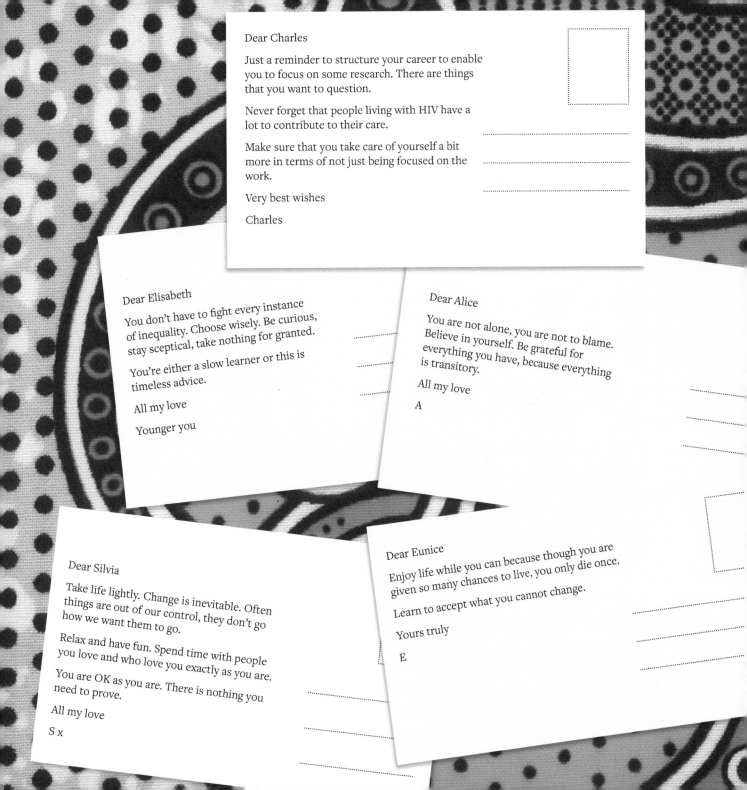

Dear Charles

Just a reminder to structure your career to enable you to focus on some research. There are things that you want to question.

Never forget that people living with HIV have a lot to contribute to their care.

Make sure that you take care of yourself a bit more in terms of not just being focused on the work.

Very best wishes

Charles

Dear Elisabeth

You don't have to fight every instance of inequality. Choose wisely. Be curious, stay sceptical, take nothing for granted.

You're either a slow learner or this is timeless advice.

All my love

Younger you

Dear Alice

You are not alone, you are not to blame. Believe in yourself. Be grateful for everything you have, because everything is transitory.

All my love

A

Dear Silvia

Take life lightly. Change is inevitable. Often things are out of our control, they don't go how we want them to go.

Relax and have fun. Spend time with people you love and who love you exactly as you are.

You are OK as you are. There is nothing you need to prove.

All my love

S x

Dear Eunice

Enjoy life while you can because though you are given so many chances to live, you only die once.

Learn to accept what you cannot change.

Yours truly

E

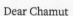

Dear Simon

It is often more effective to be diplomatic and friendly if you are trying to get people to change things – but not always.

Some things will never change unless you make a noise. If you think something is wrong or could be better, then it is unlikely to change unless people make this happen.

Appreciate people you meet because time is short – just as it was in 1987. Enjoy the opportunities you have to meet and work with inspiring people in many different countries. Always keep learning.

Please remember to chill out a bit more and not to take things so seriously.

All my love, S

Dear Chamut

Enjoy each day as it comes and play the long game! At times, the challenges of the day may seem overwhelming, or the impact you want to achieve so far out of reach. Just be patient and keep working towards your goals, because they are just around the corner.

All my love

Chamut

Dear fabulous older me

Stop eating crisps and chocolate late at night, baby, because you want to keep the 17-year-old body. Look after yourself a little bit more.

You're going to be OK. It's going to be fine. It's going to be a rollercoaster, it's going to be up and it's going to be down. There are going to be moments where you're just not going to want to be here anymore. Stick it out, because that's part of the journey. That is that is what life is about.

Even if your diagnosis was negative, you are still going to have shitty experiences in life.

You are going to have really rich and happy experiences.

Marc

PS You're a black gay man living in London. You're probably are going to get HIV at some point.

Dear Vanessa

You will find where you're meant to be and what you're meant to do, but you'll always be learning and kind, so be comfortable in that.

There are always going to be different fights, struggles and successes along the way, but no, don't struggle with that. Seek comfort in the things as they are always going to evolve and you will have a part to play in that.

Love

V

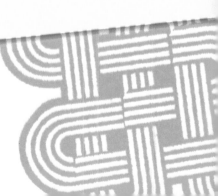

Dear Tristan

You are the most attractive now, believe in now, because you don't know the future holds or what that will be like.

Not everything will happen in the timeline that you want it to happen in. Some outcomes will be medium to long term, but you will get to be where you need to be.

If you push against something and a door is firmly shut, really think about how much energy you have to use to bash it down. Sometimes you may need to bash it down and that's OK. Remember, though, to work with doors that are already open, even if it's just a crack.

Try and be authentic. It's OK, you can play around with what that means to you, but at your core hold on to your own authenticity, as it will become easier through the rough and the smooth.

Stay true to you.

T x

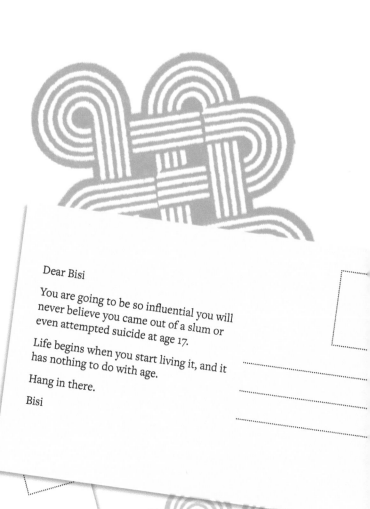

Dear Bisi

You are going to be so influential you will never believe you came out of a slum or even attempted suicide at age 17.

Life begins when you start living it, and it has nothing to do with age.

Hang in there.

Bisi

Dear Susan

Recognise your worth, listen to your inner voice and be brave. All will be well. Remember that although there's likely to be challenges along the way, remember the dark times will pass and joy is coming.

Your fabulous older self

PS Use a condom and contribute to a pension!

My darling Angelina

You will go through adversity as a young child. You will feel isolation and separation, but you will pull through and you will do well in school and in life. As you become a teen, you will face some downs, but lots of ups, too. You will make lasting friendships in primary and secondary school. Whatever the downs, don't give up. Follow your dreams, take up any and all performing arts opportunities presented to you, acting, modelling and singing and dancing. As you grow older and learn to find your place in society, keep going and believe in yourself. Don't feel that you need to conform to society. Stay true to yourself and you will go far. Make an impact. Use your voice for good, for advocacy and activism.

You will go through a challenging time in your 20s. you will receive an HIV diagnosis and all that brings, but the challenge will only make you stronger and life won't always be so terrible.

You will meet and make friends with other women living with HIV, and you will survive and thrive. You will go on to support countless other women living with HIV and your life will change for the better. You will acquire new skills, you will travel, you will change lives.

You will begin to settle into your life and to age disgracefully, something you thought you would never experience, particularly given that when you were diagnosed all you wished for was to reach the age of 30.

In later years, when you fall ill, you will pull through. Through it all, you will have a supportive network of family and friends and colleagues who will hold you up and motivate you to keep going. Together, standing on the shoulders of giants who went before you, you will all leave a lasting, positive legacy.

Keep going. Live one day at a time. Maximise your time on this earth. Enjoy and appreciate your daughter, your family, your friends. Do what pleases you. Tomorrow is not promised to any of us. Appreciate your nearest and dearest.

Live your best life, without compromise.

All my love

Angelina

(An older and more fabulous version)

Dear my younger self

First things first, you are going to make it through; through this, through everything.

No matter how terrible things seem, it is not the end of everything.

Now... right here, right now... this is your life. The way things are right now? They won't always be this way. You are bigger than the HIV virus. Do not let the virus shape who you are. Things are going to change, you are going to change; but whatever your life is in the moment, it is yours to claim. So, claim it.

Embrace the changes that your body will go through. Your boobs will sag, that tummy will grow and difficult to shed, you will get bigger everywhere. You will not understand why you are suddenly sad or can't sleep through the night without getting up three times to pee.

Feeling inadequate when you see young sexy people going on with their lives: remember you were one of them. They too will get old one day. Will they look as good as you do at your age? Time to thank your parents for those good black genes.

Own your life. Make decisions you can feel good about. Embrace the moment and make it yours. Nobody else is going to do it for you. Nobody else can think for you, love for you, or live in your place. You must do your own believing, your own forgiving, your own living.

This is how you live with little regret: you embrace everything you experience, even the things that don't feel good, because when you do that, you do what you came into this world to do – you come alive. Every up and down, every tear and thrill, this life is yours and you have no reason to apologise for who you are.

Don't apologise for figuring yourself out. You don't have to be like everyone else. You have your own place in the world, your own worth. In all the millions of ways you can be told you are not enough, don't believe even one of them. Accept yourself now, and you will be amazed at the person you become.

Accept your life now; living well with HIV and glowing in your menopause. Signs. Symptoms. Stops. Starts. Yep. This menopause tour is unique for every woman. So, for all the where-the-heck-am-I moments along the way, you are going to stumble. And you are going to learn. And you will grow and trip over your own feet long after you thought you had it all figured out. That's OK, you are not on your own.

To be alive is a precious thing. Don't forget that and don't minimise your own existence. Don't doubt how important you are, but don't take yourself too seriously, either, because nobody has it all figured out (even the ones who think they have). Everybody has scars, is afraid of something, and wants more than anything to belong.

Lastly, for now, know this: that it's never too late to be who you might have been.

Lots of love

Memory

IF I HAD A MAGIC WAND I WOULD WANT ...

Group wishes

Stigma

- A world free of HIV stigma, both crippling self-stigma and the stigma and discrimination from society and individuals.
- An end to the suffering and HIV-associated stigma.
- People to respect one another regardless of their differences; to be kind to one another and help each other as we are all fighting a silent battle within ourselves.
- Greater community involvement in the fight against HIV to get rid of stigma and that HIV becomes part of our daily conversations.
- An end to racism, homophobia and transphobia.

Religion

- All religions to be more honest and open about talking about HIV.
- Religious community leaders to stop demonising HIV and/or victimising people living with HIV.

Quality of life for people living with HIV

- More resources to support quality of life issues for people living with HIV.
- Improved and local access to help with maintaining and attaining mental health.
- Lose a bit of weight whilst being able to eat whatever I wanted and reverse any signs of ageing I have, if there's any magic left after helping the world!
- More resources and support for menopausal women living with HIV.

Treatment access, prevention and support

- A world where there is access to treatment, care and support for anyone who needs it, regardless of where they lived, who they loved or the colour of their skin.
- All children with HIV to have access to treatment regardless of where they live.
- Treatment, support, health and social care services that are available, affordable

and tailored to individuals' needs, with effective support for their needs outside of their physical health.

- Zero new infections, zero HIV-related deaths and zero stigma and in our lifetime.
- Science to find a cure for HIV. I still cannot predict when. Please wave that wand now.
- A suite of tools available to end HIV transmission globally.
- Scientists to speed up a vaccine to prevent HIV.

Health inequalities

- A world where we all practise ubuntu, make a difference to end inequalities, to end AIDS and ensure we leave no one behind.
- Policy-makers, programme implementers and communities everywhere to understand the pervasive, pathological and pernicious effects of inequalities and instil a relentless desire to eliminate them.
- To change the health beliefs, behaviours and attitudes of most communities in relation to HIV prevention.
- To demystify the HIV conspiracy theories and myths embedded in certain communities. Many are left behind.
- To end the outrageous health inequities both between countries and also within them that disproportionately impact on the lives of black people with HIV.
- To end gender-based violence that disproportionately affects women with HIV.

Empowerment

- To empower resistant mythologists, people with adverse concepts about HIV prevention and those who don't think HIV awareness is appropriate for their community.
- All parents to appreciate the benefits of sex and relationship education in schools, as I believe this will help evoke a meaningful change.
- Incentives to encourage early diagnosis or regular HIV testing in communities.
- People's autonomy to be protected and allowed to flourish, and for individuals to be respected so that we can all understand each other as unique, as special, as important.

- The elders to have the same courage that they prayed for us to have, the same boldness that they prayed for us to have to make it in the white man's land.
- Stronger and better leadership that is creative and not risk averse and is up for innovation.
- New, exciting young people coming through to work around, not just HIV prevention, but also HIV support and prevention in a wider context.
- To run an HIV clinic in Zimbabwe that is as well-resourced as the UK.
- Everyone to be as comfortable talking about sex as they are about talking about the weather! So many of the issues we face are because sex and anything related to sex is taboo.

Funding

- Funding for activists, in order to develop movement building, because real change comes from movements and yet movements have ongoing struggles for funding for basic core costs.
- More sustainable/long-term funding for women-led services, and the technical support and capacity building for women, and especially black women, who are most affected by HIV.
- Continued funding for long-term sustainability of grassroots organisations that provide support to those people living with HIV that makes a difference to their quality of life.
- Future commissioning intentions to provide services aiming to achieve the 2030 UNAIDS targets, and more investment in psychology and social care.

Research and the Greater Involvement of People Living with HIV

- Obligatory questions at conferences where researchers are presenting their findings: What cohort of women were involved in this research? How were people with HIV were involved in forming this research?
- People living with HIV to be meaningfully involved in all aspects of service design, implementation, research, monitoring and evaluation.

ACRONYMS

ABC policy	Abstain, Be faithful, use Condoms
AHERF	African Health Research Forum
AHPN	African Health Policy Network
AIDS	acquired immune deficiency syndrome
ART	antiretroviral therapy
ARV	antiretroviral
AZT	azidothymidine
BASHH	British Association of Sexual Health and HIV
BHIVA	British HIV Association
CHIVA	Children's HIV Association
DDI	didanosine, sold under the brand name Videx
GIPA	Greater Involvement of People Living with HIV
GRID	gay-related immune deficiency
HAART	highly active antiretroviral treatment
HIV	human immunodeficiency virus
MSM	men who have sex with men
NAHIP	National African HIV Prevention Programme
PCP	pneumocystis pneumonia
PrEP	pre-exposure prophylaxis
TASO	The Aids Support Organization Uganda
THT	Terence Higgins Trust
U=U	Undetectable=Untransmittable
UKC	Coalition of People Living with HIV (ceased 2007)

ORGANISATIONS

4M Mentor Mothers network
www.4mmm.org

AIDS Coalition to Unleash Power (ACTUP)
www.actupny.org

ActionAid International
www.actionaid.org

ActionAid Uganda
www.uganda.actionaid.org

African Women's Health Forum
www.africanwomenforum.org

African Health Policy Network (was African HIV Policy Network) (AHPN)
www.ahpn.org.uk

African Health Research Forum (AHERF)
www.afrehealth.org

AIDSMAP
www.aidsmap.com

British Association of Sexual Health and HIV (BASHH)
www.bashh.org

BHA for Equality
www.thebha.org.uk

British HIV Association (BHIVA)
www.bhiva.org

Big Up
lgbthistoryuk.org/wiki/Big_Up

Body & Soul
www.bodyandsoulcharity.org

Catwalk4Power
www.positivelyuk.org/2018/01/10/catwalk-power-resilience-hope/

Catholics for AIDS Prevention
www.caps-uk.org

Center for Disease Control
www.cdc.gov

Children's HIV Association (CHIVA)
www.chiva.org.uk

European AIDS Clinical Society (EACS)
www.eacsociety.org

Ffena (within AHPN)
www.ahpn.org.uk/ffena

Fast Track Cities
www.fasttrackcities.london

George House Trust
www.ght.org.uk

GMFA
www.lgbthero.org.uk/pages/category/gmfa

Global Network of People Living with HIV (GNP+)
www.gnpplus.net

HIV i-Base
www.i-base.info

International Network of Religious Leaders Living and affected by HIV (INRELA+)
www.inerela.org

International Community of Women Living with HIV (ICW)
www.icwglobal.org

Joyful Noise Choir
www.madtrust.org.uk/project/naz/

MAC AIDS Fund
www.comicrelief.com/partners/mac-aids-fund-uk

Mildmay UK
www.mildmay.org

Momentum Trust
www.momentumtrust.com

Networking HIV & AIDS Community of Southern Africa (NACOSA)
www.nacosa.org.za

National AIDS Trust (NAT)
www.nat.org.uk

National Association of People Living with HIV Australia (NAPWHA)
www.napwha.org.au

National HIV Nurses Association (NHIVNA)
www.nhivna.org

NAZ
www.naz.org.uk

OXAIDS
lgbthistoryuk.org/wiki/OXAID

Public Health England (PHE)
www.gov.uk/government/organisations/uk-health-security-agency

Portuguese League Against AIDS
www.igacontrasida.org

Positive East
www.positiveeast.org.uk

Positively UK
www.positivelyuk.org

Royal College of Obstetricians and Gynaecologists (RCOG)
www.rcog.org.uk

S.A.F.E. Kenya
www.safekenya.org

Salamander Trust
www.salamandertrust.net

Sophia Forum
www.sophiaforum.net

STOPAIDS
www.stopaids.org.uk

Tackle Africa
www.tackleafrica.org

The Aids Support Organization Uganda (TASO)
www.tasouganda.org

Terrence Higgins Trust (THT)
www.tht.org.uk

UK-CAB
ukcab.net

Joint United Nations Programme on HIV and AIDS (UNAIDS)
www.unaids.org/en

World Health Organization (WHO)
www.who.int

WHO Sexual and Reproductive Health
https://srhr.org

STUDIES

MAYISHA II Study

Sexual behaviour and HIV infection in Black Africans in England: Results from the Mayisha II survey of sexual attitudes and lifestyles

https://researchportal.ukhsa.gov.uk/en/publications/sexual-behaviour-and-hiv-infection-in-black-africans-in-england-r

NATSAL

National Surveys of Sexual Attitudes and Lifestyles

www.sciencedirect.com/science/article/pii/S0140673613619479

Nourish-UK

The Nourish-UK study aims to understand how new mothers or birthing parents living with HIV decide how to feed their newborn babies.

www.phc.ox.ac.uk/research/health-experiences/Nourish_UK

PARTNER study

A study of HIV serodifferent couples (one HIV positive and one HIV negative) to precisely estimate the risk of within couple transmission through sex during periods where condoms not used, and the positive partner was on HIV treatment.

www.ucl.ac.uk/global-health/research/z-research/partners-people-art-new-evaluation-risks-partner-study

At a Glance: HIV in Kenya (Avert)

www.beintheknow.org/understanding-hiv-epidemic/data/glance-hiv-kenya

ACKNOWLEDGEMENTS

We would like to thank all those who encouraged and supported us throughout the process of putting this book together. Especially, those who shared their stories and reflections, and trusted us to do them justice. This book would not have happened without your contributions.

We also extend our special thanks to:

Mark Santos, Executive Director, Positive East for your guidance, leadership and unwavering support on this project; Dr Michelle Croston for your time and expertise as an author and helping us through the writing process; Dr Kirsten Jack for the creative writing workshops to sharpen our writing skills and to create poems; Dr Laura Waters for your encouragement and enthusiasm about the book; and to our families and friends for your unconditional love, which gave us the confidence to see the book idea to fruition.

This project has been made possible with the provision of a financial grant from Gilead Sciences Ltd.

Thank you to Terrence Higgins Trust and Fast Track Cities Initiative London for financial assistance and support. Thanks to Positive East for hosting the project.

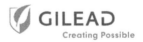

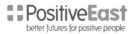

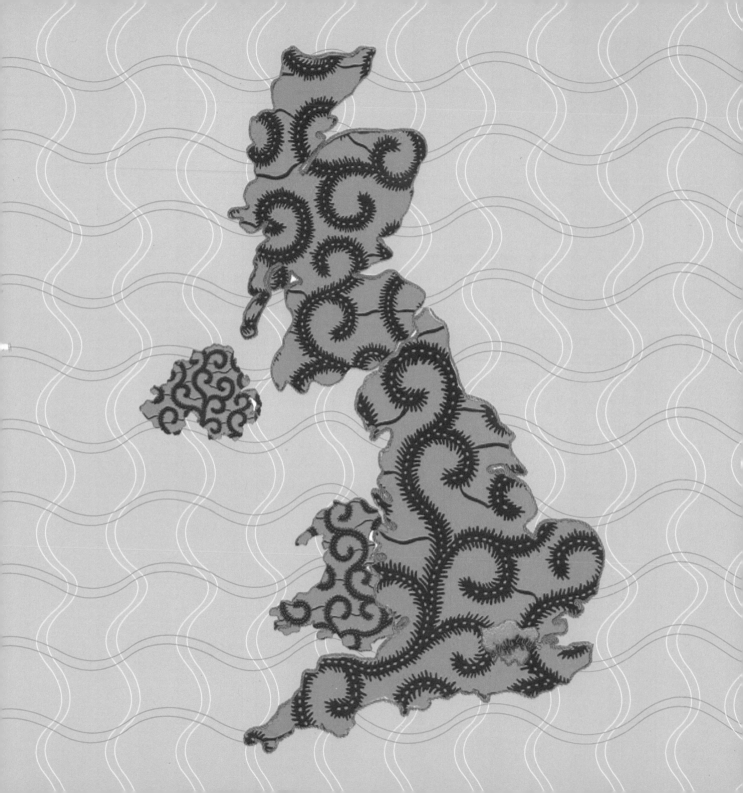